A DIET
FOR
LIFETIME
HEALTH

THE NO NONSENSE LIBRARY

NO NONSENSE HEALTH GUIDES

Women's Health and Fitness
A Diet for Lifetime Health
A Guide to Exercise and Fitness Equipment
How to Tone and Trim Your Trouble Spots
Stretch for Health
Unstress Your Life
Calories, Carbohydrates and Sodium

NO NONSENSE FINANCIAL GUIDES

NO NONSENSE REAL ESTATE GUIDES

NO NONSENSE LEGAL GUIDES

NO NONSENSE CAREER GUIDES

NO NONSENSE SUCCESS GUIDES

NO NONSENSE COOKING GUIDES

NO NONSENSE WINE GUIDES

NO NONSENSE PARENTING GUIDES

NO NONSENSE HEALTH GUIDE®

A DIET FOR LIFETIME HEALTH

Featuring the Stanford University Guide to a Healthy Heart

By the Editors of
Prevention® Magazine

Longmeadow Press

Notice

This book is intended as a reference volume only, not as a medical manual or guide to self-treatment. It is not intended as a substitute for the medical advice of physicians. The reader should regularly consult a physician in general, and particularly for any symptoms. If you suspect that you have a medical problem, we urge you to seek competent medical help. Keep in mind that exercise and nutritional needs vary from person to person, depending on age, sex, health status and individual variations. The information here is intended to help you make informative decisions about your health, not as a substitute for any treatment that may have been prescribed by your doctor.

A Diet for Lifetime Health

Copyright © 1987 Rodale Press, Inc. All Rights Reserved.

Cover Art © 1987 by Rodale Press

Published April 1987 for Longmeadow Press, 201 High Ridge Road, Stamford, CT 06904. No part of this book may be reproduced or used in any form or by any means, electronic or mechanical, including photocopying, recording, or by any information storage and retrieval system, without permission in writing from the publisher.

Library of Congress Cataloging-in-Publication Data

A Diet for lifetime health.

    (No-nonsense health guide)
     1. Nutrition. 2. Heart—Diseases—Diet therapy. 3. Cancer—Diet therapy.
I. Prevention (Emmaus, Pa.)   II. Title: Stanford University guide to a healthy heart.   III. Series. [DNLM: 1. Cardiovascular Diseases—diet therapy—popular works. 2. Diet—popular works. 3. Diet Therapy—popular works. WB 400 D5646]
QP141.D495   1987   613.2   87-4129
ISBN 0-681-40133-8   paperback

Special thanks to Eric Rinehimer for compiling and editing the information in this book.

Book design by Acey Lee and Lisa Gatti
Illustrations by Susan Rosenberger
No Nonsense Health Guide is a trademark controlled by Longmeadow Press.

2   4   6   8   10   9   7   5   3   paperback

Contents

You Are What You Eat—The Evidence Mounts

In 1979, United States Surgeon General Julius M. Richmond, M.D., announced that the next great breakthrough in health would not be a medical discovery but rather millions of individual breakthroughs as people learned to adopt healthier lifestyles. Hundreds of other physicians had the same idea at just about the same time. The critical importance of diet in controlling heart disease—the number one killer in modern society—had finally become evident. Then in 1982, the National Academy of Sciences of the United States proclaimed that cancer, too, might be very substantially reduced if people ate more wisely.

But today's food shopper is confronted by literally thousands of choices, and with this new freedom of dietary choice have come new responsibilities.

Many foods can deceive us. Garden vegetables may reach the modern table stripped of major vitamins *and* minerals—and impregnated with harmful amounts of sodium that we can barely taste. Beverages that look like fruit drinks may be concocted from sugar, caffeine and chemicals—with not a molecule of fruit to the gallon.

People worry about "junk foods," so sugary confections are disguised as "energy bars" and "granola" products. Would you put six teaspoons of sugar in a cup of milk? In the modern dairy department, they call it "low-fat" fruit yogurt.

Whereas lack of food was once the major underlying cause of illness and death, an excess of certain kinds of foods is now considered a major contributing factor to heart disease, cancer and many other diseases. Yesteryear's "poor-man's foods"—the coarse brown bread, the barley and oats, the beans and potatoes—are exactly what we today need to be eating *more* of. Evidently there is something in them that the heart likes, and cancer doesn't.

In choosing a diet for lifetime health, knowledge is power. In this book you will gain power that will give you new control over the way you feel, the way you look, the way you perform. You'll learn not only how to avoid the hidden traps in modern foods but also how to find the hidden *benefits*—the top-drawer nutrition and bargain-basement calories. You'll also learn which foods help our bodies resist illness and achieve maximum vitality.

The Top 25 Superfoods

There was a time when the phrase *health food* conjured up the image of a meager meal that didn't taste any better than grass and dust.

Today, healthy foods have taken on a whole new meaning. No longer little-known foods available only in health food stores, they're foods fresh from the supermarket and produce stand—superfoods that medical researchers believe really may make us healthy.

The researchers' evidence? Healthy people like the Eskimos, whose snacks of whale blubber should make them prime candidates for heart disease before 40 but whose fish diet actually seems to protect their hearts from harm; Italy's Neapolitans, whose high-fiber, low-fat natural foods keep them fit; and the Seventh-day Adventists, a group composed largely of vegetarians who serve up a menu for long life.

There's evidence from the laboratory, too. Did you know that there is a substance in cabbage and its clan that actually may "trap" cancer-causing agents in your body before they do any harm? Or that carrots, rich in beta-carotene, can decrease your risk of lung cancer? Or that something called a protease inhibitor, found in seeds, beans and rice, may actually be an antidote to the cancer-causing effects of a high-fat diet?

A Shopping List for Good Health

Like medical researchers, we turned to the laboratory and to healthy people when we put together our own well-balanced menu of superfoods. We also filled in with some of the foods, such as liver, oysters and green and red peppers, that Mother Nature blessed with a variety of nutrients. To make shopping easier, we included foods that, with perhaps one exception, you can find in any supermarket. And now we offer them to you with a toast: To your health!

Amaranth.   You might not find this little-known grain on your market shelves—yet. Amaranth is a food of the future. It is literally manna to millions of malnourished people in the Third World because it is remarkably high in protein and lysine, an essential amino acid—far higher than any other cereal grain. It also contains significant amounts of iron and magnesium. And it's versatile. You can use its leaves in salad and its seeds for breakfast cereal or snacks or to make flour for baking.

Bananas.   The banana disputes the old theory that if something tastes good it can't be good for you. Bananas are a great-tasting source of potassium, vitamin B_6 and biotin, another B vitamin. A medium banana contains about 100 calories, making it a delicious snack or dessert for dieters.

Beans.   If you don't know beans about beans, consider this: In several tests on patients with high blood lipids (a risk factor for heart disease), a bean diet brought down cholesterol and triglyceride levels significantly, with no serious side effects. Beans are also high in magnesium, a good heart mineral, and the B vitamins thiamine, B_6 and riboflavin. They're also an excellent nonmeat source of iron.

Bran.   One researcher calls wheat bran "the gold standard" against which the other brans, like oat and corn, are measured. Well, these days the other two are measuring up just fine. In a study of the effects of bran on constipation, corn bran was found to be therapeutically superior to wheat bran, probably because corn bran is 92 percent fiber while wheat bran is 52 percent fiber. Another group of researchers, at the University of Texas Health Science Center, also found in a feeding study with rats that corn bran cereal, even though it contained sucrose, helped prevent cavities.

And, in studies done by James Anderson, M.D., and associates at the Veterans Administration Medical Center in Lexington, Kentucky, oat bran has been found to lower cholesterol by as much as 13 percent.

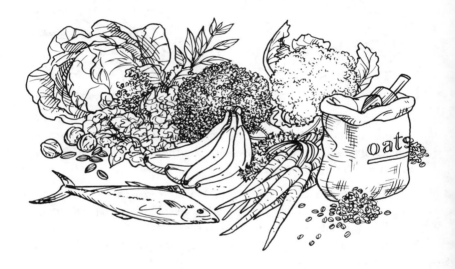

The cabbage patch clan.   Include broccoli, brussels sprouts and cauliflower in this happy family. They all figure prominently in the anticancer diet prescribed by the National Academy of Sciences a few years ago. They all appear to have some cancer-fighting properties, including vitamin A. And a cooked stalk of broccoli alone has all the Recommended Dietary Allowance (RDA) of A and twice the RDA of vitamin C, another cancer fighter, as well as calcium and potassium. Cabbage, brussels sprouts and cauliflower contain a substance that has been shown to "trap" certain carcinogens before they do any damage to the body. University of Minnesota researcher Lee Wattenberg, M.D., found that these vegetables enhance a natural detoxification system in the small intestine that keeps the carcinogens away from susceptible tissues.

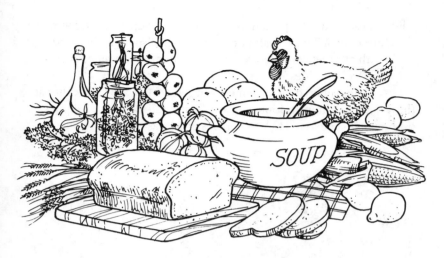

Carrots. Carrots are very high in beta-carotene, a precursor of vitamin A that is associated with a decreased risk of cancer. Carrots are high in fiber and low in calories, and even the crunch is good, toning and strengthening the gums.

Citrus fruits. A group of Florida researchers noticed an interesting statistic. Residents of southeastern Florida, many of whom have backyard citrus trees, have a lower incidence of colon and rectal cancers than people in the northern parts of the nation. The scientists at Florida Atlantic University in Boca Raton believe the secret is in the fruit. They say the vitamins A, C and E and pectin fiber have a synergistic effect: working together, they may prevent cancer.

Fish. Holy mackerel! Would you believe you could lower your blood pressure and cholesterol and triglyceride levels by eating mackerel and salmon? Researchers worldwide have discovered that certain types of fish—those containing eicosapentanoic acid, a fatty acid—protect against heart disease. They were tipped off by the healthy hearts of Greenland Eskimos, whose diet is otherwise high in fat. Apparently, it's a special kind of fat, which researchers at the Oregon Health Sciences University say may be "metabolically unique" and useful in controlling other fats that can clog the bloodstream.

Garlic and onions. These two may be bad for your breath, but they're wonderful for the rest of you. A spate of studies found that these odoriferous roots can lower cholesterol, and their oils inhibit tumor growth in laboratory experiments. Onions have been used to slow down platelet aggregation, or clumping, which can lead to deadly blood clots.

Herbs and spices.   Before you throw away your salt shaker and sugar bowl, consider refilling them—with herbs and spices. They're actually more flavorful substitutes. A couple of dashes of curry powder on fresh roasted nuts or popcorn and you'll never miss the salt. And as for sweets, a panel of tasters for the American Spice Trade Association gave rave reviews to desserts and beverages flavored with spices instead of sugar and other sweeteners. They even loved blueberry shortcake sweetened with fruit juice and cinnamon, as well as creamy custard with reduced sugar and a surprising bay leaf added for sweetness.

More Foods Worth Space in Your Pantry

Your mother—and the National Academy of Sciences—insisted you eat your leafy green vegetables. Here's why you should.

Kale, spinach and the leafy greens.   Greens like spinach contain chlorophyll, a substance that helps plants turn sunlight into food. Chlorophyll also has been found to lower the tendency of cancer-causing agents to cause genetic damage to your body's cells. Spinach and the other greens also contain significant amounts of vitamin A and calcium, although their oxalic acid content can change calcium into an indigestible compound in the body. Kale, on the other hand, has far more calcium than oxalic acid, so it's a good source of this bone-strengthening mineral.

Liver.   Usually found smothered in another superfood, onions, beef liver contains almost every nutrient going. It's rich in iron, zinc, copper, vitamins A, E, K and B_{12}, thiamine, riboflavin, biotin, folate, choline and inositol. Who can ask for anything more?

Melons.   Cantaloupes and honeydews are low-calorie treats or high-energy breakfast sources of vitamin C. One two-inch wedge of honeydew, for example, has only 49 calories but supplies more than half the RDA of vitamin C.

Nuts.   You can consume a considerable portion of your minimum daily requirement of zinc during an afternoon snack if you're snacking on nuts. Nuts, especially cashews and almonds, are very high in this trace mineral so necessary for cell growth. But don't go nutty with nuts. Zinc notwithstanding, you're also munching a handful of calories, so enjoy them in moderation.

Oysters.   Legend has it that oysters are an aphrodisiac. We don't make any claims for that, but oysters are high in zinc, shown to be necessary for proper prostate and sexual function and sperm motility. Oysters are also rich in calcium, iron, copper and iodine. But a word of caution that we rarely give about anything else: Don't eat them raw. If they're not cooked, oysters tend to pick up bacteria that can make you ill.

Peppers.   Which has more vitamin C, an orange or a pepper? Better bet on the pepper. One of these gorgeous green beauties contains twice the vitamin C of an orange.

Poultry.   Let's talk turkey—and chicken, while we're at it. They're low in calories, low in fat and high in essential nutrients and taste. An average half chicken breast contains 25.7 grams of protein, just 5.1 grams of fat and only 160 calories. With that you get a side order of vitamin A, riboflavin and niacin, not to mention iron. A chicken leg contains only 88 calories and 3.8 grams of fat. Turkey is equally good news. Three ounces of light meat without skin totals 150 calories, 28 grams of protein and 3.3 grams of fat, with respectable amounts of B vitamins.

Seeds.   High in zinc and protein, seeds (such as pumpkin, sunflower and sesame seeds) also contain something called a protease inhibitor, which seems to help protect us against cancer. Protease inhibitors have been shown to prevent liver, mammary and colon cancer in cancer-prone laboratory animals.

Note: Some people with diverticulitis may not be able to eat seeds; they are not digested well and may even block the intestine. These people should be especially wary of nuts, popcorn, strawberries, raspberries, figs, grapes with seeds, poppy seeds and caraway seeds.

Soup.   It's not only good food, it's the food that makes you eat less. A study that analyzed the food diaries of 90 patients determined that those who ate soup more than four times a week ate fewer calories a day and lost more weight than those who didn't eat as much soup. In fact, the researchers found, a soup meal contained an average of 54.5 percent fewer calories than a nonsoup meal.

More "Health" Foods from the Supermarket Shelf

Time was, foods like soybeans and sprouts could be found only in special, out-of-the-way stores. Today they're as easy to locate as sweet potatoes.

Soybeans.   They're good protein—as good as animal sources, say nutritionists at the Massachusetts Institute of Technology. They lower cholesterol, say researchers at Washington University School of Medicine. And there's some indication that soybeans are cancer fighters. Like seeds, soybeans contain protease inhibitors. And soybean products like tofu (bean curd) and miso (soybean paste) tested by researchers in Tokyo seemed to inhibit potential carcinogens called n-nitrosamines in the stomach.

Sprouts.   They're more than just a grassy accoutrement to salad and sandwiches. Studies show that the ascorbic acid (vitamin C) in some sprouted seeds and beans increases 29- to 86-fold after germination! Mung bean sprouts are especially high in magnesium and calcium. But the best news concerns the wheat sprout. It's been shown to inhibit the genetic damage to cells caused by some cancer-causing agents.

Sweet potatoes.   These superfoods deserve to appear on the dinner table at times other than Thanksgiving and Christmas. Besides being tastier than white potatoes (which are not related), they're high in vitamin A, the substance that makes carrots such a potent cancer fighter. Sweet potatoes are also low in calories. One five-inch potato contains only 148 calories.

Wheat germ.   The B vitamin thiamine is abundant in only a few foods. One of them is wheat germ, which is also rich in vitamin B_6. This versatile food was once relegated to the breakfast table, but it is now being used in everything from breads to salads.

Whole grains.   Writer Henry Miller once said, "You can travel 50,000 miles in America without once tasting a piece of good bread." But that was a generation ago, when the only place you could get a piece of good whole grain bread was at the health food store or in the kitchen of a wise, healthy cook. Whether they're in bread, cereal, side dishes or casseroles, the whole grains are the way to go. They're an excellent source of dietary fiber, suspected of protecting us from everything from cholesterol to cancer. And one Welsh study found that people who ate whole meal bread were less likely to die from cerebrovascular disease (high blood pressure and stroke).

Yogurt.   African Masai warriors consume large portions of fermented cow's milk daily, which makes their already low cholesterol levels drop even lower. In the United States, fermented cow's milk is marketed as yogurt and appears to have a similar effect on American cholesterol levels. When 26 people in a study at Vanderbilt University went on a diet of whole- and skim-milk yogurt, their cholesterol levels dropped significantly. Rich in calcium and all the nutrients that are available in a glass of milk, yogurt is also easier to digest for people who are intolerant to plain milk.

Safeguard the Nutrients in Your Vegetables

Steaming is the best way to cook vegetables in order to lose the least amount of nutritional value. When you steam a vegetable, no part of it touches the water, so you lose less nutrients. It also cooks quickly, and you use no fat at all.

Boiling, for example, destroys 57 percent of the vitamin C in asparagus and 67 percent in broccoli; with steaming, only 22 percent and 21 percent are lost. The loss of protein, minerals and other vitamins is also considerably less with steaming than with boiling.

Stir-frying is much better than skillet frying. It cooks vegetables quickly, safeguarding their nutrients, and it saves calories because it uses less oil than regular frying.

Feast on the Good Fish

In 1985, the *New England Journal of Medicine* generated national headlines when it published three major studies linking fish consumption to a decreased risk of heart disease.

The provocative articles once again focused attention on the Greenland Eskimos, for whom heart disease is rare. The Eskimo diet has been plumbed and probed since 1855, when a researcher named Rink braved the inhospitable north-country cold to make a statistical survey of their favorite foods. Though by then it included such European delicacies as bread and sugar, the Eskimo diet, as it does today, consisted almost entirely of high-protein, high-fat foods such as whale, seal and salmon.

By all rights, these Eskimos ought to be prime candidates for coronaries and strokes before their forties, but they aren't. Besides their remarkably low incidence of heart disease, they don't have the skyrocketing blood cholesterol levels that in Westerners lead to atherosclerosis (a buildup of fat deposits in the arteries), a condition responsible for one out of every two deaths in the United States. In fact, a Greenland Eskimo is almost as likely to die of a nosebleed as of a heart attack.

Saved by a Fatty Acid

One reason for this enviable good fortune may be eicosapentanoic acid (EPA). It's what's known as an omega-3 fatty acid, and it's plentiful in the oily, cold-water fish the Eskimos love.

Studies, including those reported in the *New England Journal of Medicine,* found that EPA may lower blood cholesterol considerably— even more than polyunsaturated fat does. It also triggers a major drop in triglycerides, another blood fat linked to heart disease.

This remarkable substance also reduces platelet aggregation (clotting) in the blood. Because the minute, sticky disks known as platelets are so crucial to the ability of the blood to clot, Eskimos who overdo on EPA can indeed die of a nosebleed. But in moderate amounts, EPA may cut down platelet aggregation just enough to protect against the coronary artery blockage that can lead to heart attacks and strokes.

Scientists at Oregon Health Sciences University in Portland recently found that adding fish oil to the diet decreased blood cholesterol by 27 to 45 percent and triglyceride levels by 64 to 79 percent in patients with a condition that caused their blood fat levels to shoot far above normal. (The same researchers previously produced slightly smaller drops in normal volunteers.) For some of these afflicted people, the only previous dietary treatment available was to cut dietary fats to between 5 and 10 percent of their total calories. The typical American diet contains about 40 percent fat, so the treatment is radical and difficult for most people to maintain on a long-term basis.

Interestingly, fatty fish such as salmon had usually been a strict no-no on these therapeutic diets. The researchers suggest that instead it might be a useful—and healthy—addition.

An Ounce of Fish Is Worth a Pound of Protection

A group of researchers in the Netherlands, who studied a group of middle-aged men in the industrial town of Zutphen for 20 years, discovered another fish connection. Mortality from heart disease among those men who ate—on the average—only a little over an ounce of fish a day was 50 percent lower than among those who didn't eat fish.

What is most interesting about this study is the small amount of fish that apparently exerts such strong protection. The average Dutch man eats far less fish than a typical Greenland Eskimo—less than 2 ounces compared with about 14 ounces a day—and much of it is not as rich in EPA. "This would imply," the researchers suggest, "that tiny amounts of eicosapentanoic acid have a preventive effect against coronary heart disease, assuming that eicosapentanoic acid is the only active component of the fish diet."

Another possibility, they suggest, is that there are other, as yet unknown, constituents of fish that are protective. Encouraged by their

Your Omega-3 Catch of the Day

Seafood	Omega-3 Fatty Acids (g./3½ oz.)	Total Fat (g./3½ oz.)
Salmon, Chinook, canned	3.04	16.0
Mackerel, Atlantic	2.18	9.8
Salmon, pink	1.87	5.2
Tuna, albacore, light, canned	1.69	6.8
Sablefish	1.39	13.1
Herring, Atlantic	1.09	6.2
Trout, rainbow (U.S.)	1.08	4.5
Oyster, Pacific	0.84	2.3
Bass, striped	0.64	2.1
Catfish, channel	0.61	3.6
Crab, Alaska king	0.57	1.6
Perch, ocean	0.51	2.5
Crab, blue, cooked, canned	0.46	1.6
Halibut, Pacific	0.45	2.0
Shrimp, different species	0.39	1.2
Flounder, yellowtail	0.30	1.2
Haddock	0.16	0.66

SOURCE: Adapted from *Journal of the American Dietetic Association,* vol. 69 and 71.

findings, they concluded that adding "as little as one or two fish dishes a week" could reduce heart-attack risk.

While you're unlikely to get a doctor's prescription for mackerel or salmon, they are two of the tastier and most EPA-rich fish you could add to your weekly menu. (For the omega-3 fatty acid value of different types of seafood, see the accompanying table.) Even if you're not a fish lover, the following recipes should help you prepare one or two meals a week that can do as much for your taste buds as they do for your heart. These delectable treats were created by the staff of the Rodale Food Center.

Marinated Salmon Steaks

Serve with lightly steamed asparagus.

5	cardamom pods	1⅓	pounds salmon steaks,
1	allspice berry		about 1 inch thick
2	cloves garlic, minced		lime slices (garnish)
⅓	cup lime juice		

Remove the seeds from the cardamom pods. Pulverize the seeds and the allspice in a spice mill or a mortar and pestle. In a small bowl, combine the cardamom and allspice with the garlic and lime juice.

Arrange the salmon steaks in a single layer in a shallow baking dish, then pour the marinade over them. Let stand for 15 minutes, then turn them over and let stand 15 minutes more.

Remove the fish from the marinade, then broil or grill for 5 minutes on each side, or until cooked through.

4 servings

Variation: Bake the salmon in the marinade for 25 minutes at 375°F.

Chinese-Style Braised Mackerel

Serve with Chinese rice noodles.

¼	cup rice vinegar	1	cup chicken stock
½	teaspoon low-sodium soy sauce	1	small carrot, julienned
3	thin slices ginger root	1	2 × 2-inch piece daikon radish, julienned
3	cloves garlic, halved	2	scallions, thinly sliced (garnish)
1	pound mackerel fillets		

In a glass baking dish, combine the vinegar, soy sauce, ginger and garlic. Add the mackerel, skin side up, in a single layer. Marinate for at least 10 minutes.

Bring the stock to a boil in a large frying pan. Reduce heat to simmer and add the mackerel, skin side up, and the marinade. Cover and simmer for 5 minutes. Add the carrots and radishes. Simmer for 2 to 3 minutes. With a slotted spoon, transfer the mackerel and vegetables to a serving platter.

Discard the ginger and garlic. Boil the cooking liquid until it's reduced by half, then pour it over the fish. Sprinkle with scallions.

4 servings

Herb-Stuffed Rainbow Trout

If you can't find fresh purple basil, feel free to substitute other fresh herbs.
Fennel, oregano and marjoram are especially fragrant choices.

2	whole trout (10 to 12 ounces each)	1	clove garlic, minced
¼	cup white wine vinegar	½	teaspoon Dijon mustard
2	tablespoons lemon juice		freshly ground pepper
1	teaspoon oil	12	purple basil leaves
2	teaspoons snipped chives		thin lemon slices (garnish)
1	teaspoon minced fresh purple basil		purple basil leaves (garnish)
1	teaspoon minced fresh rosemary		

Clean the trout well, leaving the heads intact. Wash with
cold water and dry well. Place side by side in a glass baking dish.

In a small bowl, mix the vinegar, lemon juice, oil, chives,
minced basil, rosemary, garlic, mustard and pepper. Pour the
marinade over the trout. Cover and marinate 30 minutes, turn-
ing the fish after 15 minutes.

Coat the broiler pan with nonstick spray. Transfer the fish to
the broiler pan, reserving the marinade. Wrap the tails with foil to
prevent burning.

Gently bruise the whole basil leaves with a spoon to release
their flavor. Place 6 leaves inside each trout, then brush the fish
with marinade.

Broil 4 inches from the heat for 3 to 4 minutes. Turn the fish
over, brush with marinade, and broil for 3 to 4 minutes more,
until light brown. Garnish with lemon slices and basil leaves.

4 servings

Salmon with Dill Sauce

Fish

¼ cup cider vinegar
¼ teaspoon Dijon
       mustard
4   4-inch pieces fresh dill
       (seed heads)
4   salmon steaks, about 1
       inch thick
1   green pepper, sliced
       into thin rings

1   tomato, thinly sliced
1   scallion, minced

Sauce

½ cup low-fat yogurt
4   teaspoons Dijon
       mustard
2   teaspoons minced fresh
       dill

To make the fish: In a glass baking dish, combine the vinegar and mustard. Add the dill and salmon and marinate for 10 minutes. Turn the salmon over and marinate for 10 minutes more.

Preheat oven to 375°F.

Cut four 8 × 8-inch sheets of aluminum foil. For each serving, place a salmon steak in the center of a piece of foil, then arrange the peppers, tomatoes, scallions and dill decoratively on top of the fish. Drizzle with marinade. Fold and pinch foil to seal the fish inside. Bake for 15 to 20 minutes.

To make the sauce: In a cup, combine the yogurt, mustard and dill.

Remove each portion of fish from its foil wrapping and serve with sauce.

4 servings

Oyster Stew

Serve with whole wheat dinner rolls and a salad of spinach and walnuts.

1	pint oysters with liquid (about 2 dozen)	1½	cups diced potatoes
3	tablespoons water	3	sprigs parsley
½	cup minced celery	1	bay leaf
⅓	cup minced onions	½	teaspoon dried thyme
⅓	cup minced leeks (white part only)	1½	cups skim milk
⅓	cup minced mushrooms	1	tablespoon lemon juice
2	cups fish stock or chicken stock	¼	teaspoon paprika
		¼	cup thinly sliced scallions (garnish)

Remove the oysters from their liquid and rinse them, rubbing lightly to loosen grit and sand. Place in a strainer to drain. Strain the oyster liquid from the container through cheesecloth and reserve.

In a 4- or 5-quart saucepan, bring the water to a boil. Add the celery, onions, leeks and mushrooms. Cover the pan and steam the vegetables over low heat for 5 minutes or until soft, stirring occasionally.

Add the stock and potatoes. Tie the parsley, bay leaf and thyme in a piece of cheesecloth and add it to the pan. Bring to a boil, then reduce heat, cover and simmer for 10 minutes, or until potatoes are tender. Remove the cheesecloth bag.

Add the oysters, along with the oyster liquid, milk, lemon juice and paprika. Heat gently for about 5 minutes. (Do not boil.) Sprinkle with scallions before serving.

4 to 5 servings

Fresh Tuna Poached in Miso

Serve with a salad of shredded daikon radish and carrots, sprinkled with rice vinegar.

2	cups chicken stock	1	pound tuna steaks, about 1 inch thick
¼	cup rice vinegar	10	ears baby corn, halved
1	tablespoon red-barley miso	1	red onion, sliced into rings
1	clove garlic, halved	1	tablespoon minced fresh parsley (garnish)
3	thin slices ginger root		
¼	teaspoon coriander seeds		

In a large frying pan, combine the stock, vinegar, miso, garlic, ginger and coriander. Bring to a boil, then reduce heat to simmer. Add the tuna, corn and onions. Cover the pan and poach the fish for 8 to 10 minutes.

Remove the tuna from the liquid with a slotted spoon and arrange on a serving platter. Arrange the corn and onions over and around the fish. Drizzle with ¼ cup of liquid. Sprinkle with parsley and serve immediately.

4 servings

Put Meat Back on the Menu

Beef's been on the grill for quite a few years now. "Eat less red meat," medical researchers have said, and we've listened. Fearful of cholesterol and fat, we've switched to more chicken and fish and heaped our salad bowls high.

And—make no mistake—you *can* eat too much meat. A diet that serves up bacon, sausage, luncheon meats, steaks, chops, hamburgers or hot dogs several times a week is a diet almost certainly too high in fat and too low in fiber to be optimally healthful.

But there's another side to the meat story. If you choose the right cuts, prepare it properly and eat it in moderation, meat can be a positively health-building food.

Facts about Fat

Consider, first of all, this question. Which has more cholesterol: beef, chicken or fish? Almost everyone gets that one wrong. The answer is that they all have essentially the same amount of cholesterol, about 75 milligrams to a four-ounce serving.

Second, the fat and calorie content of various cuts of beef and other meats varies from mammoth to surprisingly modest. Generalizations just don't work. Take a sirloin steak, for instance. Broil a six-ouncer as it comes out of a butcher's case and you've got 660 calories, including lots of fat. But trim away all the visible fat and you're left with a four-ounce steak that has only 350 calories. Fully 47 percent of the fat content has been eliminated.

Even more interesting, certain cuts of beef, such as round and flank steak, are quite lean to begin with. A broiled six-ounce round steak, untrimmed, has 440 calories. Cut away the ounce or so of fat on the steak and you're down to 320 calories and a very respectable fat level.

Don't make the mistake, though, of cooking meat *with* its fat, and trimming it off at the table. Some of the fat that melts during cooking will actually be absorbed into the meat. So trim before cooking, then broil on a slotted pan that permits some of the remaining fat to drip away. The result is good, lean, nutritious eating.

And of course, if you're cooking meat that's low in fat to begin with, you're even better off. For a list of various beef cuts and their percentage of calories from fat, see the table on page 20.

But what about *saturated* fat? Isn't beef higher in this kind of fat—believed to push cholesterol levels up—than chicken or fish? Generally, yes. But remember, generalizations can be deceiving. Choose the really lean cuts, like round, and ounce for ounce you've got a lot *less* saturated fat than we get from such common foods as stewed chicken, peanuts, cheese or even sunflower seeds.

On the plus side, beef is an extremely good source of protein, B vitamins, iron and zinc. The latter two minerals are believed to be deficient in many diets, particularly in those of women who are watching their weight.

And even a small amount of beef can greatly increase the amount of iron our bodies can absorb from grains, potatoes and vegetables. (Enter beef stew, stage right.)

However you cut it—or cook it—beef *does* have more fat than vegetables or fruits. But this is true of most protein-rich foods, including dairy products, nuts and seeds. The trick is to balance these foods with others that are extremely low in fat—fruits, vegetables, corn, rice, wheat and other grains, beans of all kinds, potatoes and pasta. Go easy

Rating the Beef *

Cut	Calories	Fat (g.)	% of Calories from Fat
Eye round	214	7	29
Chuck steak	219	8	33
Sirloin	235	9	33
Flank steak	222	8	34
Rump	236	11	40
Porterhouse†	254	12	42
T-bone‡	253	12	42
Ground beef§	248	13	47
Club steak	277	15	48
Rib eye ‖	273	15	50

SOURCES: Adapted from *Nutritive Value of American Foods in Common Units,* Agriculture Handbook No. 456, by Catherine F. Adams (Washington, D.C.: Agricultural Research Service, U.S. Department of Agriculture, 1975). *Composition of Foods,* Agriculture Handbook No. 8, by Bernice K. Watt and Annabel L. Merrill (Washington, D.C.: Agricultural Research Service, U.S. Department of Agriculture, 1975).

*Figures are based on a 4-oz. serving, trimmed of visible fat and cooked. Each cut provides about 35 g. of protein and about 4 mg. of iron, as well as about 100 mg. of cholesterol.
†Filet mignon and Chateaubriand can be included in this cut.
‡Strip loin and New York strip are synonyms for this cut.
§10% fat by weight.
‖ Delmonico and Spencer steak are synonyms for this cut.

on the butter and you wind up with a daily diet that includes meat but excludes excess fat.

A Sample Meal with Meat, and Only 25 Percent Fat

Many health authorities recommend a diet that derives no more than 30 percent of its total calories from fat. To see how that works in practice, let's begin with a well-trimmed porterhouse steak—not an especially lean piece of meat. About 42 percent of its calories come from fat. But if you include a four-ounce baked potato, one slice of whole wheat bread, four ounces of broccoli, one pat of butter and eight ounces of skim milk with your broiled steak (a four-ounce serving), you've reduced the ratio of calories from fat to 25 percent. The total calorie count for this typical dinner is a quite moderate 615.

Perhaps some comparisons with meatless dishes will help put beef's benefits in perspective:

- A macaroni-and-cheese dish, made with 1½ cups of ricotta, fontina and Cheddar cheeses, eight ounces of macaroni and 1 cup of milk, has about 45 percent of its calories tied up in fat. A flank steak, on the other hand, has only 34 percent of its calories in fat. In fact, most cuts of beef contain significantly less fat than comparable amounts of many cheeses (Brie, Gouda, Cheddar, ricotta, Swiss and Romano among them).

- A quiche made with two cups of Cheddar, spinach, rice, three eggs and one cup of light cream has a staggering 74 percent of its calories coming from fat. No wonder real men don't touch the stuff.

"Prime" Cuts Not Most Healthful

Short of taking a course in butcher-shop basics, what can a health-conscious consumer do to negotiate the meat morass? A good start would be to familiarize yourself with the meat industry's grading system. Its top rating is "prime," which means, according to the United States Department of Agriculture (USDA), that the meat is "the most tender, juicy and flavorful." What makes a prime cut flavorful and juicy is fat, not only the trimmable fat but also the marbling, the flecks of fat within the lean that are impossible to eliminate. If you purchase a prime cut, it's best to cut away the trimmable fat before cooking.

The meat industry's "choice" rating goes to cuts that don't quite have enough marbling to warrant the prime label. Still, these cuts are high in fat content and should be carefully trimmed.

Ironically, as one moves down the meat industry's rating chart, one makes a healthful ascent. The "good" and "standard" ratings are given to cuts "which lack the juiciness and flavor of the higher grades," according to the USDA. The reason? There's less fat. So you have less waste, fewer calories and less cholesterol and, perhaps best of all, the healthier cuts cost less. Fortunately, the meat industry has been offering more of the leaner cuts in the market recently.

So your choices are many. Beef's gamut runs from the cuts of the loin portion, which should be consumed in moderation and in careful balance with other foods, to the cuts of the round portion of the steer, which fall within the government's recommendation of 30 percent of calories from fat.

Breaking the Menu's Meat Code

When you eat out, however, another problem arises: identifying the cuts. While most supermarkets use standard names for the cuts of beef, restaurants use many aliases. And since there is no beef-eater's thesaurus, you need a guide. A few of the more common designations:

Chateaubriand.   This is a large tenderloin, sometimes called filet mignon. This is always at least a choice cut, and it might be prime. It cost the restaurant more to get and it'll cost you more.

Surf 'n' turf.   You can ask the waiter wishfully if this is haddock and round steak, but typically this is a shellfish (usually lobster) and a tenderloin cut of beef that by itself would be filet mignon.

London broil.   This is a flank steak and is a highly recommended cut at home or out. It'll cost you less in a market or a restaurant, and from a nutritional standpoint it is one of the best cuts of beef.

Whether you're buying meat at the supermarket or ordering it at a restaurant, be assertive. Don't feel that you're inconveniencing the meat cutter by asking him to trim fat for you. And make it clear to the waiter that the size of the tip depends on whether or not you get the beef exactly the way you want it. This allows you to enjoy beef, not only without reservation but also with the knowledge that you're doing something good for yourself.

How Fiber Helps Your Body Stay Fine-Tuned

Years ago, nutritional scientists viewed dietary fiber the way they once viewed "vitamin B": It was supposed to be a single substance with a single function that was rarely given a second thought by medical people.

But vitamin B has become B complex, and dietary fiber (the roughage of yesteryear) is now surprising a lot of people with a complexity of its own.

The American Cancer Society and the National Cancer Institute now want us to put more fiber in our diet. The food industry embraces it. The popular press hails it. And research labs around the world add support to decade-old hypotheses that it may help prevent obesity, colon cancer, heart disease, gallstones, irritable bowel syndrome, diverticulosis and diabetic conditions.

The "F Complex"—Not As Simple As Once Thought

With all this fuss, it's become clear that dietary fiber is more diverse in its forms and biological effects than anyone ever imagined.

And among medical people, fiber's potential for promoting health has never seemed greater. The F complex has arrived.

"Nowadays most nutritionists realize that dietary fiber is multifaceted," says Peter J. Van Soest, Ph.D., a leading fiber researcher at Cornell University. "They know that it's not just one thing but a collection of things—a variety of elements with a variety of functions."

This latter-day insight into fiber's true nature has already helped set aside some old ideas on the subject. False: "Bran" is synonymous with "fiber." False: All fiber is fibrous, or stringy. False: All fiber tastes the same.

The fallacies are more apparent as soon as you realize that dietary fiber is actually made up of the indigestible remnants of plant cells (mostly cell walls)—remnants that come in at least six types and show up in everything from bulgur to blueberries. (See the table on pages 26 and 27.) And the differences in physiological impact among these six classes of fiber can be as vast as that between penicillin and spring water. Here's what scientists know so far.

Cellulose. Cellulose is the most prevalent fiber and probably comes closest to the notion of what fiber ought to be. It is indeed fibrous, softens the stool and abounds in all the expected places— fruits, vegetables, bran, whole-meal bread and beans.

But you'll find it in some unlikely places, too, such as in nuts and seeds, and it does more than the old notions suggest. It increases the bulk of intestinal waste and eases it quickly through the colon. All of which means, of course, that it prevents constipation, but some investigators say that these actions also may dilute and flush cancer-causing toxins out of the intestinal tract. Research also indicates that cellulose may help level out glucose, or blood sugars, and—because of its ability to fill you up without fattening you out—curb weight gain.

One thing it can't do, however, is lower your cholesterol. That's a function reserved for other kinds of fiber.

Hemicellulose. This word is a misnomer—hemicellulose is not half cellulose. It has a chemical character all its own, but it usually shows up wherever cellulose is and shares some of its traits. Hemicellulose, too, may help relieve constipation, water down carcinogens in the bowel and aid in weight reduction. And, like cellulose, it has no known effect on cholesterol.

Pectin. This form of fiber may be better at pushing down cholesterol levels than any other kind.

"For some reason, water-holding fiber like cellulose has no influence on serum cholesterol levels," says David Kritchevsky, Ph.D., biochemist and coeditor of *Dietary Fiber in Health and Disease.* "But water-soluble fibers like pectin and gums can reduce cholesterol."

But then pectin doesn't have a celluloselike influence on the stool. It can't do a thing to deter constipation.

Just the same, researchers have been looking into the possibility that pectin can aid the elimination of bile acids through the intestinal tract, short-circuiting the development of gallstones and colon cancer. Common sources of pectin are apples, citrus fruits, grapes, berries and—contrary to fiber lore—bran.

Gums and mucilages. These are sticky fibers that you eat every day without even realizing it, for you usually encounter them as plant-derived thickening agents in everything from ketchup to store-bought cookies.

But investigators have discovered that gums, at least, can do far more than give condiments body. They've found that locust-bean gum, karaya gum, guar gum, oat gum and others can lower cholesterol significantly. And they've shown that a few gums can even help diabetics handle blood sugar better.

"There's a lot of scientific excitement surrounding the gum fibers," one researcher explained. "They seem to be more effective in the treatment of diabetics than some other fibers, and they're certainly more palatable than the water-soluble ones."

Lignin. The main talent of this form of fiber is to escort bile acids and cholesterol out of the intestines. There's even some evidence that it may prevent the formation of gallstones and may offer protection against colon cancer.

You'll find high proportions of lignin in cereals, bran, whole-meal flour, raspberries, strawberries, brussels sprouts, cabbage, spinach, kale, parsley and tomatoes. The more mature the vegetable, the greater the lignin content.

Finding the Fiber You Need

Fiber Type	Probable Functions	Food Sources	

Cellulose	Relieves constipation, counteracts carcinogens in the intestinal tract, modulates glucose, curbs weight gain.	Apples
		Bran and
		  whole grain
		  cereals
		Brazil nuts
		Brussels sprouts
		Carrots
		Lima beans
		Peanuts
			Pears
			Peas
			Rhubarb
			Whole
			  wheat
			  flour

Pectin	Lowers cholesterol, counters bile acids in the intestinal tract, offers protection against colon cancer and gallstone formation.	Apples Bananas Beets Berries Bran Carrots	Grapes Okra Oranges Potatoes
Gums/ Mucilages	Lower cholesterol, modulate glucose levels.	Dried beans Oat bran Oatmeal	

Good Sources of Fiber

But lignin, pectin, gum or some other type of fiber isn't sold in quart jars on your grocer's shelf. Nature has already packaged them in countless foods, in combinations that can produce a startling array of physiological changes. And it's these fiber foods, not the fiber types, that researchers have scrutinized the most. Here's a rundown of fact and fable concerning some of these top fiber sources.

Bran.   This flaky remnant of grains is one of the world's richest sources of dietary fiber. (Not *the* richest, because the raspberry, for one, has more fiber.) And it contains not one but several types of fiber,

Fiber Type	Probable Functions	Food Sources	

Hemicellulose	Relieves constipation, counteracts carcinogens in the intestinal tract, curbs weight gain.	Apples
		Bananas
		Beets
		Bran and
		    whole grain
		    cereals
			Green beans
			Radishes
			Sweet corn

Lignin	Escorts bile acids and cholesterol out of the intestines, offers protection against colon cancer and gallstone formation.	Bran and
		    whole grain
		    cereals
		Brazil nuts
		Brussels
		    sprouts
		Cabbage
		Kale
		Parsley
			Peaches
			Peanuts
			Pears
			Peas
			Raspberries
			Spinach
			Strawberries
			Tomatoes

SOURCES: Adapted from "Topics in Dietary Fiber," A Report of the Cornell University Agricultural Experiment Station, G. A. Spiller, ed. (New York: Plenum Press, 1978).
"Fiber Analysis Tables," A Report of Research of the Cornell University Agricultural Experiment Station, *American Journal of Clinical Nutrition*, October, 1979.

including cellulose, hemicellulose and pectin. But the generalizations about bran can stop right there, for there are too many discrete brans, each with its own makeup and functions.

Wheat bran has a reputation for relieving constipation, and research concurs (though a recent study indicates that corn bran may be even better at solving this problem). And evidence suggests that wheat bran may help modulate glucose levels in diabetics and reduce the symptoms of diverticulosis, an intestinal disorder.

A controversy is brewing, however, over whether your morning bowl of wheat bran can have a positive effect on cholesterol. Most of the evidence has said no, but the latest study on the subject begs to differ.

Investigators in Sweden added concentrated wheat bran to the diet of patients with high cholesterol levels, then monitored the effects. Surprise: The patients' low-density lipoprotein (LDL) and very low-density lipoprotein (VLDL) cholesterol (the harmful kinds) decreased slightly, and high-density lipoprotein (HDL) cholesterol (the beneficial kind) increased dramatically.

There's no such controversy, though, surrounding the cholesterol-lowering effects of oat bran. James W. Anderson, M.D., of the University of Kentucky in Lexington, has seen to that. He put oat bran on the nutritional map when he demonstrated in several studies that adding oat bran to the diet can reduce cholesterol levels drastically. In one such experiment involving men with elevated cholesterol, the reduction averaged 13 percent.

On top of that, says Dr. Anderson, oat bran is tastier than a lot of other fiber-rich fare. "Oat bran is palatable as a hot cereal and can be incorporated into muffins, breads and other prepared foods," he says.

But it would be a mistake to expect oat bran to relieve constipation. It's rich in water-soluble fiber, which generally has no effect on bowel movements.

Corn bran, however, is more versatile. It not only can ease the symptoms of constipation but also can lower LDL cholesterol, reduce the blood fats known as triglycerides and perhaps improve the body's ability to handle glucose. This latter capability was suggested by a study indicating that a daily intake of as little as 26 grams (less than an ounce) of corn bran could improve people's scores on glucose tolerance tests.

Legumes.   Peas, soybeans, lentils, chick-peas—these legumes and their kin have high fiber content, but few people realize just how high. They actually outdo most fruits and vegetables. Canned baked beans, for example, register over 7 grams of dietary fiber per 100 grams of beans (about 3½ ounces), while cooked broccoli weighs in at around 4 grams and cooked cabbage at just under 3 grams.

Much of this fiber is water soluble, which, as you might guess, makes legumes likely agents for lowering cholesterol. And research is slowly confirming this crucial capability. Dr. Anderson and a colleague, for example, discovered that they could lower serum cholesterol in men with excessive cholesterol levels by adding about four ounces of pinto and navy beans to the men's daily meals. Total cholesterol dropped a remarkable 19 percent.

"While bean-supplemented diets were as effective as oat bran-supplemented diets in lowering serum cholesterol concentrations," the investigators say, "oat bran was better tolerated [with fewer problems like intestinal gas] by our patients." But can legumes help ease the problem of constipation? Probably not. Can they help control glucose levels? Probably, especially if the legumes happen to be soybeans. Researchers have been reporting that both soy hulls and a powdered soy supplement can improve glucose tolerance.

Vegetables and fruits.   Scientists have tested very few of these for fiberlike feats, though it's obvious that these foods contain types of fiber known to do a lot of healthful deeds. Researchers instead have busied themselves with measuring the fiber constituents and total fiber content of these edibles — and overturned some misconceptions in the process.

For example, we now know that "vegetable fiber" isn't all cellulose. Often, as in the case of green beans and brussels sprouts, it's not even *mostly* cellulose. Similarly, "fruit fiber" isn't 100 percent pectin, though it usually has a high percentage of that type of fiber. Cellulose, lignin and other types are in the mixture, too.

And, as you may already know, the total fiber content of a fruit or vegetable can surprise you. The vegetables with the highest fiber ratings, for example, include sweet corn, parsnips, carrots, potatoes and peas. And among the highest-ranking fruits are raspberries, pears, strawberries and guavas. Ounce for ounce, a peach has more fiber in it than a turnip does, cherries more than a green pepper, and carrots more than cabbage.

Getting Enough Fiber

Unfortunately, there's no Recommended Dietary Allowance for fiber and very little data on optimum amounts. More and more researchers, though, are venturing some concrete recommendations based on the evidence that does exist. John H. Cummings, M.D., a noted fiber expert in England, has advocated a fiber intake for adults of 30 grams (about one ounce) a day. And other investigators have echoed this suggestion.

"We really don't know what the optimum intake of dietary fiber should be," says Dr. Van Soest. "But it is possible to get some positive

Thirteen Tasty Ways to Add Fiber to Your Diet

- Leave the peels on apples when you bake them or make applesauce.
- Roll chicken in corn bran or oat bran for oven baking.
- Add barley to vegetable soup.
- Make tostadas with beans instead of beef.
- Top yogurt with bran, sunflower seeds or chopped apples.
- Make your own breakfast granola with rolled oats, bran, raisins, slivered almonds and dried fruit.
- Use fresh, unpeeled fruit instead of fruit juice.
- Substitute beans for some or all of the meat in casseroles.
- Make taco burgers by combining lean ground beef, kidney beans, tomato paste and spices.
- Pop popcorn and munch away.
- Create desserts using fresh, unpeeled fruit like peaches and pears. Try filling unpeeled peach halves with cottage cheese and slivered almonds, for example.
- Eat potatoes with the skins on.
- Mix cooked beans into vegetable or tuna salad.

benefits from fiber at the 30- to 40-gram mark, although you have to adjust the amount to what is comfortable for your own body."

But even this amount is far more than many Americans are getting, so some authorities have been coupling their fiber recommendations with some sound advice. Increase your fiber intake slowly, they say, to give your system time to adjust, gradually incorporating a variety of fibers from a variety of naturally occurring sources.

After all, you have a vast F complex to choose from.

Better Nutrition for Kids

It's not as if a mother doesn't try. It's just that it's not always so easy when baby Billy locks his jaw every time you try to feed him what he should eat instead of what he wants. Later, when he starts elementary school, you don't know whether (and how often!) he trades his nutritious tuna on whole wheat for a triple pack of cupcakes in the school cafeteria.

How then can you possibly know for sure whether he's getting the proper nutrition—at least the Recommended Dietary Allowances (RDAs)?

Unfortunately, that question isn't all that easy to answer. But one thing seems clear: How well your child measures up to the RDA is totally up to you.

Understanding the RDA

Before you can best assess your child's nutritional health, you need to understand what the RDA is all about. Actually, there are two RDAs—the Recommended *Dietary* Allowance and the U.S. Recommended *Daily* Allowance (USRDA). The Recommended Dietary Allowance was first developed in 1943 as a guideline for establishing an adequate intake of specific nutrients for *healthy* people in particular groups based on age, sex and estimated weight. (This means anyone with a chronic illness or a metabolic disorder cannot be included in this

31

group. They could need more.) Since then the RDA has undergone periodic revisions, and today the Food and Nutrition Board of the National Research Council has established minimum limits for 13 vitamins, three minerals, nine trace elements and three electrolytes.

The U.S. Recommended Daily Allowance was established by the Food and Drug Administration for use by food manufacturers in giving nutritional information about their products on labels. Since food labels are small, there isn't enough room for the Recommended Dietary Allowance for individual age and sex groups. The USRDA merely simplifies things by using just one value—usually the highest level needed by any age group or sex group (excluding pregnant and lactating women).

Does this mean your children are expected to hit 100 percent of the Recommended Dietary Allowance every day?

"No," says Lendon Smith, M.D., an Oregon pediatrician and author of *Dr. Smith's Diet Plan for Teenagers* and *Feed Your Kids Right.* "Everyone who has any kids knows that they don't eat right every day. Even though we'd like them to, it's unrealistic to expect it. You should look at the overall diet. It's okay if your child doesn't get the RDA every day. But is he getting it every week?"

Another thing to remember is that getting less than 100 percent of a nutrient does not necessarily mean you will become instantly unhealthy. Scientifically, your intake of a nutrient isn't considered on the low side until it falls below 67 percent of the RDA, and even then a deficiency disease isn't imminent. Knowing that alone should make you feel better if your child's diet doesn't measure up for a day or two.

Nutrients in Short Supply

Not surprisingly, certain vitamins and minerals are more likely than others to be in short supply in a child's diet. One study conducted at the University of Washington in Seattle tested a group of healthy children from the ages of $3\frac{1}{2}$ to 9 to see how they fared on the RDA for vitamin C, thiamine, riboflavin, vitamin B_6, vitamin B_{12} and folate—all essential nutrients for normal childhood development. While intakes were adequate for most nutrients, some of the children showed intakes below 70 percent for folate and B_6.

Dr. Smith feels that zinc, a trace element that aids normal growth, also is often low in the average child's diet. But it's iron, more than any other nutrient, he says, that is most commonly in short supply.

Alvin N. Eden, M.D., agrees. Dr. Eden, a practicing pediatrician in New York City and associate clinical professor of pediatrics at the State University of New York, Downstate Medical Center in Brooklyn, says iron is a very neglected area. "I think there's a large group of children out there who are iron deficient without being anemic. For this reason, I think it's important for parents to consider giving their children an iron supplement. In fact, the most important thing I tell parents is to 'think iron.' "

Of course, if children would eat liver, the best source of iron, there would never be a deficiency problem. Nor would a deficiency of zinc, selenium, chromium, vitamin A, riboflavin, vitamin B_{12} and folate ever occur. Unfortunately, when it comes to liver, most kids consider going to bed without *any* supper the better alternative. (For information that will help you upgrade your children's diet, see the tables on pages 34 to 40.)

(continued on page 41)

Two Typical Menus Analyzed

There's always room for improvement, and no one knows that better than the mother of a child who prefers peanut butter and more peanut butter.

We asked pediatrician Lendon Smith, M.D., to assess a typical day's menu for two typical children—Elizabeth, age 7, and her brother, Josh, 11. Menu A, on page 34, lists Elizabeth's intake for one day. Menu B, on page 35, lists Josh's. Neither meets the daily allotment for *all* nutrients. A computer analysis reveals that both diets are on the low side for iron and zinc. Elizabeth's diet for this particular day is also low in some of the B vitamins, and Josh's falls short for vitamin A.

By making a few substitutions, adjustments and additions, Dr. Smith illustrates how easy it can be to naturally add extra nutrients to your child's diet. In fact, with Dr. Smith's revision, Elizabeth's total nutrient intake soared to over 100 percent. Josh's vitamin intake more than tripled, and his calcium, zinc and iron levels were boosted, too.

Menu A: for a Typical 7-Year-Old Girl	Dr. Lendon Smith's Improved Menu	Dr. Smith's Comments
BREAKFAST		
½ cup sugar-coated cereal with ½ cup low-fat milk ¼ cup orange juice (store brand)	½ cup Grape-Nuts with raisins and ½ cup low-fat milk 1 whole orange or ½ cup fresh orange juice	"The Grape-Nuts will provide more across-the-board nutrients (and less sugar!) and the raisins a little extra shot of this day's allotment of iron. A whole orange is more likely to have more vitamin C, bioflavonoids and fiber."
LUNCH		
1 peanut butter and jelly sandwich on a potato roll 1 package cheese and crackers 1 cup cran-raspberry juice 3 Oreo cookies 1 peanut butter cup	1 peanut butter and banana sandwich on whole grain bread Thermos of homemade soup, such as chicken noodle or vegetable 1 cup apple juice 3 oatmeal cookies Celery stuffed with peanut butter	"It goes without saying that a banana is a far more nutritious choice than jelly. Whole wheat bread might be a better choice to help give her more B vitamins. The thermos of nutritious soup will help fill a child up and help eliminate her desire for cookies and candy. Apple juice will help bolster this day's low iron allotment, as will the day's low iron allotment, as will the oatmeal cookies."
DINNER		
Baked ham (about 1 ounce) 1 bite steamed broccoli ½ cup scalloped potatoes, made with carrots and onions ¼ cup gelatin dessert with a bit of applesauce mixed in ½ cup low-fat milk	Baked ham (2 ounces) 1 spear broccoli ½ cup scalloped potatoes, made with carrots and onions ½ cup applesauce 1 cup low-fat milk	"With the exception of the gelatin dessert, this is a decent meal, although the child may have eaten more had she not had such a large lunch or so much sugary food at breakfast and lunch."

Menu B: for a Typical 11-Year-Old Boy	Dr. Lendon Smith's Improved Menu	Dr. Smith's Comments
BREAKFAST		
½ cup orange juice 2 slices 7-grain bread with peanut butter	1 whole orange 2 slices 7-grain bread with "old-fashioned" peanut butter ½ cup low-fat milk	"The fresh orange is included for vitamin C, bioflavonoids and fiber. The milk will help increase calcium. Use homemade—'old-fashioned'—spread. It doesn't contain the salt and sugar store-bought varieties contain."
LUNCH		
1 peanut butter and jelly sandwich on 7-grain bread 1 peanut butter and chocolate granola bar 1 raspberry fruit bar	1 peanut butter and banana sandwich on whole wheat bread Trail mix (dried fruit, raisin and nut mixture) Carrot sticks	"As with his sister, this boy should be weaned from jelly to a more nutritious alternative—bananas. The trail mix, unlike granola, will come a long way in improving the RDA, particularly some of the B vitamins, vitamins A and E and magnesium. The carrots will help restore this day's vitamin A supply."
DINNER		
1 slice meat loaf made with lean beef 2 new potatoes made with herb butter ½ cup peas 1 potato roll 1 cup low-fat milk	1 to 2 slices meat loaf made with extralean beef 2 new potatoes with herbs 1 stalk broccoli 1 slice whole wheat bread 1 cup low-fat milk	"A little extra meat loaf will add extra zinc and iron, which are low on this day. The butter seems an unnecessary addition of fat to this diet and adds nothing in terms of nutrition. The broccoli helps increase the calcium intake."

Recommended Dietary Allowances for Children

Nutrient	Major Functions	RDAs for Children 4–13	Comparison to Adult RDA	Good Food Sources Children Can Love
Vitamins <u>A</u>	Necessary for healthy skin, good vision and bone growth. Bolsters the body's immune system. Believed to help guard against cancer.	Ages 4-6 — 2,500 I.U. Ages 7-10 — 3,300 I.U. Boys 11-13 — 5,000 I.U. Girls 11-13 — 4,000 I.U.	Less Less Same as adult male Same as adult female	Cantaloupe, carrots, dried apricots, hard-boiled eggs, sweet potatoes, vegetable soup, watermelon
Thiamine (B₁)	Helps keep nervous system functioning smoothly.	Ages 4-6 — 0.9 mg. Ages 7-10 — 1.2 mg. Boys 11-13 — 1.4 mg. Girls 11-13 — 1.1 mg.	Less Less than adult male; more than adult female Less than young adult male; same as adult male Same as young adult female; more than adult female	Baked beans, oatmeal, rice, rye bread, sunflower seeds, whole wheat bread

Riboflavin (B₂)	Carries oxygen to body cells. Helps build healthy blood.	Ages 4-6 – 1.0 mg. Ages 7-10 – 1.4 mg. Boys 11-13 – 1.6 mg. Girls 11-13 – 1.3 mg.	Less Less Less than young adult male; same as adult male Same as young adult female; more than adult female	Almonds, cheese (particularly Brie), lean beef hamburger, low-fat yogurt, milk, wild rice
Niacin	Good for memory and moods. Helps lower levels of blood fats—cholesterol and triglycerides.	Ages 4-6 – 11 mg. Ages 7-10 – 16 mg. Boys 11-13 – 18 mg. Girls 11-13 – 15 mg.	Less Less Less than young adult male; same as adult male More than young adult female; more than adult female	Almonds, baked beans, dried dates, peanuts and peanut butter, sunflower seeds, tuna, white meat chicken, whole wheat bread
B₆	Helps keep immune system healthy and keeps blood clots at bay.	Ages 4-6 – 1.3 mg. Ages 7-10 – 1.6 mg. Ages 11-13 – 1.8 mg.	Less Less Less	Bananas, filberts, sunflower seeds, tuna, white meat chicken
Folate	Aids in normal functioning of the central nervous system.	Ages 4-6 – 200 mcg. Ages 7-10 – 300 mcg. Ages 11-13 – 400 mcg.	Less Less Same	Cantaloupe, orange juice, red beets, romaine lettuce (on sandwiches)

(continued)

Recommended Dietary Allowances for Children—*Continued*

Nutrient	Major Functions	RDAs for Children 4-13	Comparison to Adult RDA	Good Food Sources Children Can Love
Vitamins *(cont.)*				
B₁₂	Necessary for healthy blood and nerves. Guards against anemia.	Ages 4-6—2.5 mcg. Ages 7-13—3.0 mcg.	Less Same	Lamb, low-fat yogurt, milk, Swiss and Cheddar cheeses, tuna, white meat chicken
Biotin	Helps certain enzymes utilize fats, proteins and carbohydrates.	Ages 4-6—85 mcg. Ages 7-10—120 mcg. Ages 11-13—100-200 mcg.	Less More Same	Black raspberries, eggs, grapefruit, milk, oranges, turkey and chicken legs, whole wheat bread
C	Helps hold cells together. Its antiviral and antihistamine properties are believed to guard against a list of diseases, from the common cold to cancer.	Ages 4-10—45 mg. Ages 11-13—50 mg.	Less Less	Baked potatoes, blackberries, blueberries, cantaloupe, cherries, orange juice, strawberries, tomato juice

	Function	Amount	More/Less	Food Sources
D	Works with calcium to build strong bones.	Ages 4-13 — 400 I.U.	More	Egg yolks, milk, tuna (also plenty of sunshine)
E	Promotes healthy circulation by preventing formation of clots. Protects cells against oxidation. Protects immune system.	Ages 4-6 — 9 I.U. Ages 7-10 — 10 I.U. Ages 11-13 — 12 I.U.	Less Less Less	Almonds, lobster, peanuts and peanut butter, pecans, sunflower seeds
K	Essential for normal blood clotting.	Ages 4-6 — 20-40 mcg. Ages 7-10 — 30-60 mcg. Ages 11-13 — 50-100 mcg.	Less Less Less	Broccoli, cheese, milk, watercress sandwich
Minerals Calcium	Necessary for healthy bones, teeth and muscle.	Ages 4-10 — 800 mg. Ages 11-13 — 1,200 mg.	Same More	Buttermilk, cheese, ice cream, low-fat yogurt, milk, whole wheat pancakes
Iron	Essential for manufacture of red blood cells.	Ages 4-10 — 10 mg. Ages 11-13 — 18 mg.	Same as adult male Same as adult female	Chicken and turkey (white and dark meat), lean beef hamburger, molasses, raisins, sweet potatoes

(continued)

Recommended Dietary Allowances for Children—Continued

Nutrient	Major Functions	RDAs for Children 4-13	Comparison to Adult RDA	Good Food Sources Children Can Love
Minerals (cont.)				
Magnesium	Aids calcium in forming strong teeth and bones. Helps prevent kidney stones.	Ages 4-6—200 mg. Ages 7-10—250 mg. Boys 11-13—350 mg. Girls 11-13—300 mg.	Less Less Less than other teenage boys: same as adult male Same as adult female	Baked potatoes, bananas, beans, molasses, nuts, oatmeal, peanut butter, whole wheat spaghetti
Zinc	Aids normal growth. Sharpens sense of taste, smell and sight. Aids wound healing.	Ages 4-10—10 mg. Ages 11-13—15 mg.	Less Same	Chicken legs, crab, hot dogs, lean beef hamburger, oatmeal, pork chops, shredded wheat
Trace Elements Chromium	Helps insulin control blood sugar levels.	Ages 4-6—0.03-0.12 mg. Ages 7-13—0.05-0.2 mg.	Less Same	Brown rice, cheese, cornbread, goose, oatmeal, vegetable soup, whole wheat bread, whole wheat spaghetti
Selenium	Helps keep heart and muscles sound. Enhances heart health. Protects immune system.	Ages 4-6—0.03-0.12 mg. Ages 7-13—0.05-0.2 mg.	Less Same	Breads, corn on the cob, seafood, shredded wheat, tuna, whole wheat pancakes

Meeting the RDA

Not to worry. There are plenty of other ways to get your liver-shy kids to eat right. By including certain core foods in the diet each day, the doctors we spoke to say you'll be doing your best to help your children meet their RDA.

For breakfast, the most concentrated form of nutrition is a whole grain cereal and a fruit, either whole or as juice. "Hot oatmeal with applesauce and raisins tastes great and is very nutritious," says Dr. Smith. Or, for a change of taste, try serving leftovers from last night's dinner. "There's nothing wrong with a chicken leg for breakfast," he says. "It's protein."

Our experts also suggested it's best to pack a child's school lunch rather than depend on what's being served in the cafeteria. Whole wheat bread or another whole grain should always be used for sandwiches. It provides needed B vitamins. Peanut butter is just fine, but eliminate—or at least cut down on—the jelly. Instead, substitute a banana. Always include fruit in the lunchbox, too. For snacks, opt for carrot sticks or trail mix (an assortment of nuts, dried fruits and raisins).

For dinner, serve a lean meat or fish, steamed vegetables, and fruit for dessert. If you want to feed your kids pastry, think whole grains, and go for oatmeal cookies instead of brownies.

Allow your children to drink only low-fat or skim milk. "Kids shouldn't drink too much milk," says Dr. Eden. "I think milk is a little overrated. Too much spoils an appetite, and it's too high in fat to be good for you. Two glasses a day is plenty."

Is there anything else you can do?

Dr. Smith suggests giving a multiple vitamin, "for insurance, not as a food substitute. It's good to remember that the RDA is only a minimum, and an estimate at that," he says. "And keep in mind that every child is different. How each person absorbs nutrients and their degree of wellness can vary."

Living Alone and Eating Well

A popular comedienne once joked that she wanted to open a restaurant strictly for singles. Her scheme was to make them feel at home. Instead of a table, each diner would eat standing over a sink.

The image should be familiar to anyone who has ever lived alone. You know who you are. You're the ones who've made peanut butter fudge brownies for supper, eaten cold pizza for breakfast and consumed whole meals bathed in the romantic glow of refrigerator light. The closest you've ever come to owning a pet was finding something in the back of the fridge with fur on it. Was that what used to be tapioca pudding?

Needless to say, good nutrition rarely comes in single servings. If you're one of the 23.2 percent of the American population living in what the census bureau calls a one-person household, it's a safe bet your diet makes World War II C-rations look like health food.

"What do I usually eat?" says a 31-year-old single personnel consultant in Washington, D.C. "TV dinners, M & M's, Häagen-Dazs ice cream every Sunday night. I wouldn't eat this way if I weren't single.

I wouldn't be so careless. But I want you to know I've seen the error of my ways—all 20 pounds of the error of my ways."

Overweight but Undernourished

Like this reformed careless consumer, many singles atone for their dietary indiscretions only after they learn the direct relationship between their waist size and the number of disposable single-serving food packages in their trash. But the damage they do with their quickie over-the-sink meals and their fast-food feasts is far from merely cosmetic. Next to the poor, they may be the most undernourished people in America.

George Demetrakopoulos, M.D., M.P.H., is medical director of the Medical Nutrition Center of Greater Washington (D.C.). Among the patients who come to him for nutritional assessments are people who should know about nutrition: employees of several of the government's top health-regulation agencies. But, he says, it doesn't seem to give them an edge if they're single. In a study of 40 single men and women between 25 and 45, he found most were deficient in zinc, folate and vitamin B_6. The women were also deficient in calcium and were getting only 57 percent of their Recommended Dietary Allowance (RDA) of iron.

"These are not typical people," says Dr. Demetrakopoulos. "These are nutrition-conscious people. They should have performed above average, but they didn't. Imagine," he says, "the ones who are not."

Though the research is meager, it seems to show that living alone is a significant nutritional risk factor even if you're nutritionally savvy. In fact, eating for one seems to be most perilous for young single women who are aware consumers and elderly single men who don't know their way around the kitchen without a guide.

Researchers at Auburn University took a look at the diet of 50 single professional women, most of whom usually made food lists and menu plans and avoided convenience foods. Despite those good intentions, their diet was low in calories, calcium, iron, vitamin A and thiamine. What's more, their good food habits seemed to be done in by their frequent lunches out.

In a study of 3,477 people between 65 and 74, researchers at the University of California and the University of Texas found that poor men living alone had the lowest intake of milk products, fruits, vegetables, meat, poultry and fish of any group. And they were more likely to be getting less than two-thirds of the RDA of protein, riboflavin, vitamins A and C and other nutrients.

What makes singles turn to meals of tea and toast, or worse? Busy schedules, dieting, lack of motivation or cooking skills, and even loneliness and depression can contribute to many a meager mealtime, say the experts. And unfortunately there's usually no immediate retribution for a bad diet that might persuade a fast-food aficionado to change his ways.

"Most nutritional problems don't manifest themselves right away, so it's easy to cheat," says David Ostreicher, D.D.S., professor of nutrition at Bridgeport University in Connecticut, who is single. "If you're not getting enough vitamins A and C, you might not know until 20 years later when you develop cancer. If you're eating a diet high in saturated fats and salt—the staples of most convenience foods—you might not know until you have your first heart attack at age 50."

Eleven Steps to Nutritional Bliss

The problem thus stated, what do you do? "Get married," jokes Dr. Demetrakopoulos. Or, failing that, simply steal some tricks from your wedded friends who are following a better diet.

Cook for four.   "Never, never cook for one," says Dr. Ostreicher. "Cook for four, eat one serving and freeze the rest in individual servings. You'll be making your own convenience foods, you'll pay less and you will be eating better."

Make shopping lists.   "All my married friends have lists; none of my single friends do," says Dr. Ostreicher. Why a list? First, it will make you plan your weekly meals. And it will keep you from straying into dangerous territory: the family pack of cookies that looks too good to pass up, 500-calorie-a-slice frozen pizza and the special on heavenly hash ice cream. Needless to say, don't go shopping when you're hungry and, advises Dr. Ostreicher, have regular shopping days so you aren't tempted to dash into the deli for a hot pastrami on the way home because there's nothing in the fridge.

Shop with a friend.   Going on the premise that everything is better with a friend, try shopping on the buddy system. Your companion will be your conscience. "If you have a companion, you can discuss what you're going to buy and make with the other person," says Dr. Demetrakopoulos. "Alone, you'll wind up buying things you'd be better off without."

Steer for the freezer section.   Many singles have given up on fresh vegetables because they are forgotten and then grow moldy in the refrigerator before the week is up.

"Psychologically, that stops you from buying vegetables the next time," says Dr. Ostreicher. "But right next to the frozen convenience foods you'll find plastic bags of vegetables with nothing added that are just as nutritious as fresh. You can reseal the plastic bags so you can use what you like and freeze the rest. You don't pay more and they don't give you all that excess salt and fat."

Don't buy big.   Those family packs and mammoth cans may be cheaper, but they're no bargain if you have to throw half of the food away. If you want to buy the bigger packages, consider sharing them with a friend. And if you see a cut of meat or produce you like in a larger package, ask a store employee to repackage it.

Develop good eating habits.   If you have to, pretend you're eating with a friend. Would you eat a chicken leg over the sink or swig milk right out of the bottle if you had a dining companion? Then don't do it when you're alone. "Always set the table," says Dr. Ostreicher. "You decide how—with a tablecloth or place mats. Candlelight might be excessive, but get into the habit of having a place setting, even if you're just grabbing a piece of fruit.

"That stops the noshing. When you live alone, you often get into the habit, when you've got nothing to do, of standing in front of the open refrigerator and snacking. Always eat at the table, always with a place setting."

Make eating for one an experience.   Lynn Shahan, author of *Living Alone and Liking It!* says that during her first year of eating alone she became "a pretty skinny kid" because mealtime, so often spent with family and friends, lost its appeal. Her solution for happier soloing at the dinner table was to buy new and interesting foods and experiment with recipes so eating became more of an adventure.

Don't eat all your meals alone.   Have friends or neighbors in for dinner. Start a cooking club with your fellow singles. Call your local agency on aging to find out if your neighborhood provides free or low-cost meals for older people at community centers or churches.

Or join a group like Single Gourmet, a New York-based organization that tackles the problems of eating alone by arranging for up to 100 singles to eat out together seven to ten times a month.

Cofounder Art Fischer says it will not only improve your social life and your outlook, it may also improve your digestion. "Doctors have told us that one of the problems with single people eating alone is they not only eat all the wrong food, they eat too fast, which can cause digestive problems," says Fischer, whose group numbers 3,000 members in the New York metropolitan area. "In a group like ours, you'll spend two to three hours eating a meal that, if you ate it alone, would be gone in a matter of minutes. People tell us that they've never been able to eat garlic before without getting indigestion, but when they eat it at a Single Gourmet dinner, it doesn't bother them at all. Really, it's the single lifestyle that doesn't agree with them."

The psychological boost of having pleasant companions and good food is inestimable. "One is a very lonely number," says Effie Seaman, a writer who joined Single Gourmet after the death of her physician husband. "This gives you a reason to get dressed and go out, wearing your finery, which is far better than sitting in front of the TV with a sandwich."

Eat out wisely.   Ned Schnurman, executive producer of the acclaimed PBS television series *Inside Story,* regards eating out "as a form of theater."

"Eating is one of my principal interests. I eat out 300 nights a year," says Schnurman, who is in his midfifties and single. By all logic, Schnurman should be as wide as he is tall. Instead, even with his rigorous restaurant schedule, he managed to lose 25 pounds in the last few years. How? He eats out wisely. When he chooses a dinner spot to please his palate, he adjusts his other meals accordingly. A light breakfast and lunch are the perfect preludes to the "good saloon fare" he favors: simply grilled chicken, fresh vegetables and "a little wine—very little." He avoids heavy sauces and bypasses the dessert cart for fruit. "I don't think it matters where you eat," says Schnurman. "Even if you eat out as much as I do, you can make sure you're eating things of good nutritive value."

Choose light fast-food fare.   "It's a real break for singles that most fast-food restaurants now have salad bars," says Dr. Ostreicher. "But if you want to have a burger, have a plain burger. Don't order the fancy burger with the special sauce. And especially don't order a cheeseburger." Almost 90 percent of the calories in cheeses and special sauces come from fat.

Consider supplements.   "People will not make drastic changes in their diets, so I recommend supplementation," says Dr. Demetrakopoulos. Most women need calcium, he says. And most of the patients he has tested don't get even a third of the RDA of zinc (15 milligrams). But most single people are going to have to face up to it: A bad diet can't be rescued by pills entirely. "Going to the trouble of taking supplements when your diet is grossly inadequate," he says, "is like having a nicely painted house with no windows."

CHAPTER
SEVEN

New Eating Skills for Once-and-for-All Weight Control

"Ninety percent of weight-loss programs fail because they *don't* tackle behavior," says Henry Jordan, M.D., director of the Institute for Behavioral Education in King of Prussia, Pennsylvania. But what happens when they do? That's exactly what Rita Yopp Cohen, Ph.D., of the department of psychiatry at the University of Pennsylvania, wanted to find out. She reviewed the results of several weight-loss studies and, not surprisingly, those that involved behavioral techniques came out on top. One particular study compared the weight loss of 102 women who had undergone one of three treatments: behavior therapy, drug therapy or a combination of drug and behavior therapy. At the end of six months the women taking diet pills lost an average of 32 pounds and the combined-treatment group lost an average of 34 pounds. By contrast, the behavior therapy women lost only 24 pounds.

But researchers found a striking reversal of the treatment results at a one-year follow-up. Behavior therapy patients "regained far less weight"—4 pounds—while the women who had taken the diet pills regained 18 pounds and the combined-treatment group regained 23½ pounds, almost three-quarters of the weight they had lost. At the end of one year, the net weight loss of the behavior therapy group was the greatest.

This study is typical of many that show that weight loss through behavior modification is slower than with other methods. But, like the tortoise and the hare, slow and steady wins the race.

Ronette Kolotkin, Ph.D., director of the behavioral/psychological component of the Dietary Rehabilitation Center at Duke University Medical Center, has been working with obese patients for years. "It's not always the pattern, but among my most successful patients are some who didn't lose weight for the first two or three months on the program," she says. "Some actually gained weight. But eventually they lost 50 to 60 pounds over the course of two years. It's a lifetime change we're talking about—not a fast solution."

"If you have dieted in the past," says Gerard Musante, Ph.D., a behavioral psychologist who directs a weight-loss clinic in Durham, North Carolina, "you must ask yourself, why didn't it work? Primarily, it's because what you wanted was a magic formula—and there is no such thing. With those shortsighted methods you become obsessed with how much you weigh: The scale becomes a deity to which you pay homage."

"The truth is, some overweight people are looking for structure," says Kelly Brownell, Ph.D., a behavior specialist at the University of Pennsylvania. "A rigid diet offers structure, yes, but with impermanent results. Behavior modification offers a structure to behavior— with lasting results. Eventually, the person who loses weight through changing his behavior and restructuring his lifestyle will gain a sense of control."

To help you get started on your plan of control—to reform your own attitude about food once and for all—we talked to the nation's top behavior modification experts about their most successful techniques. Here are seven tips that they recommend.

Keep a Food Diary

Imagine a salesperson without an appointment book. Or executives who don't write down the meetings they have to attend. In fact, think of any busy person trying to successfully meet the responsibilities and challenges of the day without some kind of written record. It would be next to impossible!

Well, weight loss is a challenge, too. You have to know what you're eating and what you plan to eat. And the best way to do that is to keep an accurate record—a food diary.

At the University of Pennsylvania obesity clinic, Dr. Brownell and his colleagues, Albert Stunkard, M.D., and Thomas Wadden, Ph.D., put a great deal of emphasis on the diet diary. "The food diary serves a number of very valuable functions," explains Dr. Brownell. "I know people who have kept a food diary for ten years. It can get to be a nuisance, but almost all of our patients, after they've lost weight, tell us later that the food diary was the most useful tool of behavior modification. I'm not saying that you have to keep a diary for ten years—although those people who did tended to maintain a good weight loss. There are many, many people who keep a food diary for a while and eventually quit keeping it once they've begun to do well on the program."

What does keeping a food diary entail? Basically, it means writing down everything you eat every day and at what time you eat it. Most of the top behavior modification clinics in the country encourage people to elaborate even more. "We have people write down everything they put into their mouths—along with when they ate it, with whom, what mood they were in, how hungry they felt, the degree of appetite and so on," says Maria Simonson, Ph.D., director of the Health, Weight and Stress Clinic at Johns Hopkins University Hospital in Baltimore. "At the end of two weeks—even without being on a diet—they've usually lost one to three pounds."

No diet, no diet pills—just a record of you and food. How can such a simple device work? It works in several ways, the experts say. First of all, it makes you aware of how much you're actually eating. According to Isobel Contento, Ph.D., an associate professor of nutrition and education at Teachers College, Columbia University, studies show that "people who eat a lot tend to underestimate the amount of food they eat, while people who eat a little tend to overestimate the amount of food they eat," she says. "When it comes to food intake, it is difficult to be accurate."

Aside from sheer quantity, a diary points up the quality of foods you eat. If breakfast is often a cup of coffee and a doughnut, lunch is a hamburger and a soft drink, dinner consists of a small salad followed by a bowl of ice cream, and a late-night snack means pretzels or potato chips, the dieter can be reminded in black and white that this kind of diet is definitely lacking in good nutrition.

Even so, our experts say you should never divide food into categories of "good" and "bad." Dr. Brownell explains, "In our program, there are no forbidden fruits, no foods that the dieter must *never* eat. Saying 'I'll never eat cake again' sets the dieter up for failure when they 'succumb' to having a piece at someone's birthday party. Eating something that's a no-no in the dieter's book will lead to self-blame and a sense of having failed again in a weight-loss attempt."

At the University of Pennsylvania clinic, the focus is on limiting calories at a healthy level—one where the dieters can still enjoy their favorite foods, but with an eye to optimum nutrition. "We ascribe to nutritional principles above all," Dr. Brownell says. His colleague Dr. Wadden puts it this way: "The idea is not to deprive yourself of the foods you crave, but to be able to control yourself when faced with those foods."

A food diary also can reveal essential personal truths about your eating patterns—not just preferences for certain foods but also times of the day or days of the week (such as the weekend) when you tend to overeat or eat out of sheer habit.

"By seeing your eating patterns," says Dr. Simonson, "you can eliminate some unnecessary eating. For example, the diary may show a person that he's eating a snack every afternoon even when he doesn't really feel hungry."

A diary can also help detect some psychological reasons behind your overeating. You may notice, for example, that you overeat every single time you have lunch with your mother. You love her dearly, but somehow seeing her transports you back to the days of "Clean your plate or you can't have dessert."

Discovering your personal eating patterns through the pages of a diet diary is a major step you can take toward your goal of permanent weight loss. It will help you understand why you overeat. Your diary can serve as your "personal warning system" to tip you off *before* your eating gets out of control. Once you have taken this step, the next one, becoming the master of your own eating habits, will come more easily.

Discover Your Food Cues

How often do you go into the kitchen and fling open the doors of the cabinet underneath the sink—the one where all the cleansers are—just for the heck of it? Most likely, you hardly ever do. Now how many times do you walk into the kitchen, fling open the refrigerator door and mindlessly snatch something from the shelf? Well, you don't have to answer that one. You probably get the point. The refrigerator is one of those food cues, something that signals a behavior in you that makes you want to eat, whether you planned to or not. To gain control over your eating behavior, you need to cultivate new habits and strategies to cope with "the enemy."

For example, let's see what you can do to deal with the refrigerator. Obviously, one answer would be to have two refrigerators—one that you could put out of the way, perhaps in the cellar, that would contain items of temptation like ice cream or soft drinks. (This, of course, is assuming that you keep these items because someone else in the family wants them. If they're for you, you should throw them away.) Unfortunately, most people don't have this option. So here's where a little strategy comes in.

Load the front of the refrigerator with fruits, vegetables and meat-and-potato-type leftovers. The half-eaten lemon chiffon pie should be pushed way in the back and hidden from view. The storage shelves on the inside of your refrigerator door should be restricted to holding items like eggs and butter. As for the freezer compartment, put ice cream or similar snacks in the back—behind the frozen meats and vegetables and completely out of sight. The old adage, "Out of sight, out of mind" can work quite well with your appetite.

Stage and television actor James Coco, who lost 110 pounds while attending Dr. Musante's North Carolina clinic, Structure House, credits his success to being able to pin down several of his danger traps. "I found that whenever I talked on the telephone, I munched on nuts," he recalls. "There was always a bowl of them next to the phone. At parties, I always found myself next to the buffet table. And I ate incredible amounts of food while I was cooking—I love to cook. It took wearing a surgical mask to break me of that habit!"

Behavioral therapists refer to control over eating cues as "stimulus control and environmental management." Here are some of their most useful recommendations.

- Make eating a "pure" experience. Eat only at the kitchen table or dining room table, and always use a place setting. Never eat in any room other than the kitchen or dining room. And never eat while standing up. (Remember the refrigerator habit?) Also, says Dr. Stunkard, "avoid pairing your eating with other activities." Many an extra calorie is added by eating while reading, watching TV, walking, driving, cooking and so on.

- Shop wisely. The "out of sight, out of mind" adage works well here, too. If you don't buy it, you won't be tempted to eat it.

- Store food wisely. Keep food only in the kitchen and pantry. Place high-calorie items in hard-to-reach places, on the highest shelves or behind other foods in the refrigerator. Put the cake saver away with the pots and pans until you need it. (Seeing it empty may spur you to fill it.) And don't use glass jars to store brownies—fill the jars with herb teas and dried beans instead.

- Make use of signs—whatever works for you—on the refrigerator, your desk or wherever necessary.

- Be on guard at social gatherings. "When people are in social situations—when they're happy and celebrating and feeling particularly gregarious—they may overeat, especially if they've been having alcohol," says Dr. Wadden. "Alcohol decreases our inhibitions, which include our inhibitions toward eating." Dr. Wadden suggests eating something *before* you go to the party, such as a salad or a light sandwich. He also recommends making the first drink a glass of water. That way you won't be so hungry or thirsty soon after you arrive.

Conquer Calories with Complex Carbohydrates

This food group has had a dirty reputation with the overweight for years. Baked potatoes were frowned at, and spaghetti drew sneers.

But now complex carbohydrates are being introduced into weight-loss schemes. In fact, they have become positively welcome as scientists increasingly report their helpfulness in moderate programs of weight loss. It turns out that the butter and rich sauces that get ladled onto the complex carbohydrates are the real villains in the calorie department.

Complex carbohydrates, particularly the unrefined kind, offer us filling, stomach-satisfying bulk as well as nutritive value.

Develop New Eating Skills

Old habits die hard. They seem chiseled into our personality by years of repetition, as much a part of us as our skin. And bad eating habits are no exception. You try to change them, but before you know it, they've snagged you again—you're in their power. The only way to conquer them is to square off, look 'em in the eye, see them for what they really are and pull a few fast ones before they get you first.

When breaking bad eating habits, it's best to meet them on their own turf—at the table. Here are some new skills to practice so that eating doesn't get out of hand. They're very simple, yet extraordinarily effective.

Slow down! It was another one of those "sneaky" experiments. Fifty-five women who had lost weight through behavior modification and 26 women who had never gone through such a program were told they would be entering a "tasting room" to rate the flavor of three different crackers. But behind a one-way screen was a group of researchers who were there to observe the real purpose of the experiment: to see how much each woman would eat in a seven-minute period. As the researchers anticipated, the women who had learned their eating habits through behavior modification ate less than the women who hadn't. This observation leads to an interesting insight into the weight-loss story. It suggests that *eating less is associated with eating slowly.*

Experts feel that, in general, overweight people eat faster than people of normal weight. And there are plenty of overweight and formerly overweight people who can attest to that.

Eating slowly is a technique with a particularly nice side effect: It allows you to savor food. In his book, *I Almost Feel Thin,* Dr. Stunkard quotes one of his patients, a young college woman who had struggled with overeating for years: "A couple of nights ago, when I was studying, I went into my roommate's room and took a cookie, just *one cookie,* from a box that she had there. I ate it very slowly, chewing it carefully and tasting every part of it. And then I went back in my room to study. I was in absolute awe of myself—was this the same Mary O'Brien who two months ago wouldn't have been able to stop at *ten cookies,* let alone one; who would have eaten the whole box and then another one if it were there?"

But how do you learn to eat slowly when you have spent your life chowing down as if you were in a pie-eating contest? Our experts recommend these three tips:

1. Chew food *thoroughly* before swallowing.
2. Count each mouthful of food and lay your fork or spoon down after every bite.
3. Be the last to start eating and the last to finish. "When you are eating with other people, talk, rearrange your napkin, cut your meat into tiny pieces—stall any way you can to be the last person to start eating," says Dr. Brownell. "During the meal, maintain a pace that will guarantee that you are the last one finished."

Think about it. If eating is to be a pleasurable activity, it deserves your time and concentration.

Stick to your own plate.   Many overweight people are compulsive plate cleaners—and they don't stop at their own plate, either. In a house where there are young children (who are notorious for their erratic eating patterns), parents sometimes get into the habit of "picking" at their children's leftovers. For a person prone to weight gain, this can be a dangerous practice. A roll of plastic wrap kept in a very handy place (perhaps even on the table) will help solve that problem: Simply wrap the plate and put it in the refrigerator—immediately. Or give it to the dog. Whatever you do, don't leave it on the table.

Aside from laziness (that is, avoiding stashing leftovers because it requires effort), the reasons behind plate cleaning often stem from guilt feelings that go back to childhood. James Coco recalls, "Before I began to deal with behavior modification and changing my lifestyle, there never was a leftover in my house. I really was the sort of person who would go gung-ho and clean out the cupboards and the refrigerator and then wake up at 2:00 in the morning, find nine peppercorns and eat them. And I realized it had something to do with growing up Italian, and also being told at the table, 'Finish your food—people are starving all over the world,' and I'd think, 'Oh, my God, I can't let people starve. I'd better eat my food.' And one day I realized that people were still starving—but I was getting fat."

Leave a bit behind. It may sound like heresy, but to break yourself of compulsive plate cleaning, practice leaving food on your plate. Some successful weight reducers say they now leave just a mouthful—as a matter of course. Also, learn to police your own portion control by dishing out your meal from the stove directly to the plate. If some family members want seconds, all they have to do is go back to the kitchen. Serving food "family style," with all that extra food heaped into serving bowls on the table, only encourages latent plate cleaning, experts say.

Plan and Preplan

There's something very satisfying about the ritual of eating a nice meal at the table. Eating ravioli right out of the baking pan while standing next to the kitchen sink may provide a pleasant taste experience, but somehow something is missing.

It's not surprising that some behavioral therapists blame haphazard, unplanned eating as a primary cause of overweight. Dr. Musante's strong belief in structured eating is what led him to call his clinic Structure House. Structured eating is breakfast, lunch and dinner— the meals we take to fulfill our basic nutritional needs. Anything beyond that he considers *un*structured.

After 12 years of research, working with hundreds of patients, Dr. Musante and his staff came to the conclusion that every episode of unstructured eating is the result of one of three things: habit, boredom or stress.

Eating out of habit rather than hunger is quite common, says Dr. Musante, because it is an automatic response—something we learned in childhood.

Boredom, however, is a little more insidious. "As soon as people gain weight, they stop doing things," he says. "They've decreased the repertoire of behaviors they can engage in; they're limited in the ways they can entertain themselves." But they know that one way they can still entertain themselves is with food. Because they have nothing to do, or because they don't want to do the things they liked to do when they were thin, they eat.

In the stress situation, Dr. Musante says, people use food as a tranquilizer. "You're upset, you eat, you feel better. What it all comes down to is changing a lifestyle that is characterized by habit, boredom and stress."

At Structure House, one way employed to get people to make these changes is by getting them in the habit of planning all their meals well in advance. "We're not saying you can't engage in unstructured eating, but that if you do, be aware of it," says Dr. Musante.

How far in advance are we talking about? Many people find that planning their meals about a week in advance works the best. It also helps to buy only as much food as you'll need for each meal.

Erase Black-and-White Thinking

By now you know how important it is to be careful of what you're eating when you're trying to lose weight. But there's another dictum for dieters that's equally important: Be careful of what you're *thinking.*

"One of the most damaging patterns of thinking is on-and-off thinking—what I call black-and-white thinking," says Dr. Wadden. "The biggest problem dieters have is they have such high expectations of themselves that they can't possibly meet these expectations." The result: They abandon the diet.

"They're not so much perfectionists, but rather people who buy into the body image promoted by the media—they buy into the thought that they should be thin," he explains. "A lot of people think that if they don't achieve their goal, anything short of the goal is a failure. It's a very dichotomized thinking pattern: You've either succeeded or you've failed. We try to help people quantify success and say if you lost 2 pounds that it's terrific. It wasn't the 2½ pounds you had your heart set on, but it's still a great success."

Overeating in itself does not lead to negative feelings, explains Dr. Brownell. It's how a person *perceives* the overeating that matters the most. For example, there are some overweight people who would respond to eating an extra-large piece of cheesecake with this range of thinking: "Oh, what a pig I am; I'm so disgusted with myself I don't deserve to lose weight." Dr. Brownell calls this a catastrophic statement—a value judgment that leads to negative feelings.

"However, there are all kinds of ways to look positively upon events—even overeating," he says. A statement such as, "Well, that was an extra 300 calories. I'll have to take a nice, long walk after dinner tonight to make up for it," works much, much better.

So how can you stop being so down on yourself? One way is to state your feelings out loud. It helps show how silly they really can be. Dr. Wadden says this works well in his weight-loss clinics. "In a group session, for instance, one person says to herself and the others, 'I really screwed up badly last night. I ate 100 calories of potato chips above what I said I was going to eat. I feel like a failure.' Then I might say to a member of the group, 'Would you please tell her she's a failure because she ate too many potato chips?' When the group harangues her, it sounds ridiculous, and we end up laughing."

Putting all this into practice isn't easy at first. You've got to give it time. "In behavior modification," says Dr. Brownell, "you must realize first that the changes won't come overnight. It takes a lot of practice to get over those negative thoughts and feelings that have occurred many times."

Pick a Partner

Making an event more interesting or fun is a lot easier when it involves more than one person. The same goes for dieting. While it may be stretching it a bit to say dieting is fun, it's sometimes a task that's a lot easier to tackle if there is someone around for support.

Diet experts say the support can come from anyone—a fellow dieter, a friend at work or a spouse. For some people a support group is the answer.

"Of course, there is no rule that applies to every person," says Dr. Brownell, who wrote a book on the subject, *The Partnership Diet Program.* "For some people it helps to enlist the aid of a spouse; other people find that they need to get away from home—to a clinical setting—to break the cycle of overweight.

"Eventually, though," he says, "most people find it easier to lose weight and keep it off if the environment they live in supports their efforts. That's why spouses are important. They can make it easier to comply with the program of behavior modification. They help reinforce the technique of the weight-loss program."

Sugar Highs and Lows

Feeling down in the dumps? Before you head for the doctor, head for the kitchen. Maybe that cabinet full of cookies, candy and cola is what's fueling your bad mood.

Lester I. Tavel, M.D., D.O., Dr.P.H. (doctor of public health) believes that large amounts of sugar in the diet can be an emotional downer.

"Too much sugar causes an increase in insulin in the body, and the result is low sugar," he says, adding that this may lead to such symptoms as depression, nervousness and weakness.

He suggests that a modified diet can stop these symptoms. "I recommend that the patient moderate his sugar intake, perhaps drastically, depending on the patient."

Dr. Tavel adds that further dietary changes may also help to improve mood. He recommends increasing the amount of complex carbohydrates in the diet, as well as increasing protein consumption.

While changes like these may seem drastic, the benefits far outweigh the adjustment required—and those benefits include not only greater emotional stability but also possible weight loss.

CHAPTER
EIGHT

The Stanford University Guide to a Healthy Heart

From the Stanford University Heart Disease Prevention Program

Artificial hearts, coronary care units, heart transplants, bypass surgery—these are the widely publicized remedies for America's cardiovascular epidemic, a modern plague of heart attacks, strokes and other woes that kill over a half million people each year.

But is this technology all that stands between you and coronary doom?

Let's hope not. Though these methods have certainly saved lives, they are most often merely plugs in a dike that's been crumbling for a lifetime. They are the eleventh-hour antidotes to a malady that usually begins decades before the first telltale chest pains or heart attack.

The main cause of heart disease is atherosclerosis, a slow buildup of cholesterol and fatty tissue in the arteries. Like pipes corroding secretly through the years, your arteries narrow and harden as the buildup increases, restricting blood flow and making you feel old before your time. Typically, by middle age you have thick, rough deposits clinging to the artery walls, like so much lime in subterranean tunnels. And when the arteries supplying blood to the heart muscle narrow to

60

about two-thirds their normal diameter, you may have a heart attack. And when the blood supply to the brain is choked off, you may have a stroke.

But the good news (which has yet to claim as much media attention as the high-tech treatments) is that, in almost everyone, atherosclerosis can be prevented and perhaps to some extent even reversed. In fact, 80 to 90 percent of strokes and heart attacks can be prevented. Thanks to research at California's Stanford University and around the world, we now know that atherosclerosis is caused largely by factors entirely within our control.

The three most dangerous factors are high blood cholesterol, high blood pressure and cigarette smoking—each capable of single-handedly doubling or tripling your risk of heart trouble. Lack of exercise, over-

Stanford: A Crossroad of Expertise

The Stanford Heart Disease Prevention Program is a national crossroad of expertise in the study and prevention of cardiovascular diseases. Since 1971 its wide spectrum of scientists and other professionals has been working to discover what causes and prevents heart disease—and put that information to work in thousands of lives. Program researchers have conducted pioneering studies in exercise physiology, weight control, smoking cessation, blood fats and cholesterol and the effects of health education on community health practices. The program is part of the Stanford Center for Research in Disease Prevention.

Staff members include John W. Farquhar, M.D., director; Nathan Maccoby, Ph.D.; Peter D. Wood, D.Sc.; Stephen P. Fortmann, M.D.; William L. Haskell, Ph.D.; June A. Flora, Ph.D.; C. Barr Taylor, M.D.; Byron W. Brown, Jr., Ph.D.; Prudence Breitrose; Joel D. Killen, Ph.D.; Robert Superko, M.D.; Michael J. Telch, Ph.D.; and Paul T. Williams, Ph.D.

weight and stress are three others that can tip the odds against you. In combination, these six can work a kind of dark synergism, with each risk factor compounding the treachery of every other.

The risk factors shorten life. Eliminating the risk factors extends life. Indeed, the recent decline in death rates for heart disease is due less to advances in medical technology than to reductions in risk factors.

Here's why—and how—you can dramatically reduce your chances of encountering America's number one killer.

Eating to Live

The verdict as to whether cholesterol contributes to heart disease is final. The scientific community has duly investigated, indicted and convicted cholesterol not merely of being associated with heart disease but of *causing* it.

A panel of physicians and scientists convened by the National Institutes of Health proclaimed, "Elevated blood cholesterol level is a major cause of coronary-artery disease. It has been established beyond a reasonable doubt that lowering definitely elevated blood cholesterol levels . . . will reduce the risk of heart attacks due to coronary heart disease."

This finding is backed by a long line of research, including the Coronary Primary Prevention study by the National Heart, Lung and Blood Institute. In this massive trial, in which Stanford and ten other research centers participated, 3,806 men with high cholesterol were monitored for ten years as they took daily doses of either a cholesterol-lowering drug or a placebo (inactive substance). The men were also asked to keep their intake of dietary cholesterol at moderate levels. The result was that the rate of heart disease in the treated men was 19 percent lower than in the placebo group.

The study revealed that for every 1 percent drop in blood cholesterol, there is a 2 percent decrease in risk of heart disease. And, as the results imply and later analysis of the data confirmed, this drop in risk can be achieved through either drugs or diet—preferably diet.

Consume less cholesterol, fat, salt and sugar.   Only about 5 percent of people may require drugs to keep their cholesterol levels down. The rest of us, fortunately, can eat our way to decreased cholesterol levels—and decreased risk. It's mostly a matter of gradually moderating our intake of two kinds of foods: those containing cholesterol itself and those containing saturated fat, which also increases cholesterol in the bloodstream. But cholesterol isn't the only dietary foe of the heart. There's also salt—the familiar guest at most American dinner tables and a close associate of high blood pressure. Several studies, including research at Stanford, have shown that salt can contribute to high blood pressure and that even moderate cutbacks in salt intake can ease blood pressure down. Certainly your body needs salt, but only about a quarter of a teaspoon a day. The average consumption in the United States is 20 times that amount.

Scientists also suspect another beloved staple: sugar, a simple carbohydrate. In some cases it can dramatically boost the liver's production of very low-density lipoprotein (VLDL) cholesterol, an especially dangerous type. And because sugar is packed with "empty" calories, it can easily nudge out more nutritious foods in your diet and—worst of all—increase your chances of obesity, a top coronary risk factor.

Eat more vegetables, beans, grains and fruit.   The dietary opposites of sugar—complex carbohydrates (vegetables, beans, cereal grains and unprocessed fruits)—are comparatively low in calories, fat and cholesterol and high in vitamins and minerals. They are therefore the perfect substitutes for foods loaded with cholesterol, saturated fat, salt or sugar. Besides that, because complex carbohydrates are relatively low in calories for their bulk, they can fill you up without loading you down with extra calories. Researchers have already demonstrated that, despite what some dieters believe, diets high in complex carbohydrates can help you lose weight.

Fiber up.   Foods high in complex carbohydrates contain what has become one of the great nutritional discoveries of the past few years: fiber, the indigestible but crucial remnants of plant foods. Researchers have linked high-fiber diets with low rates of heart disease and cancer of the colon, rectum and breast. And there's evidence that certain fibers (including those in beans, oats, carrots, apples and other fruits but excluding wheat bran) can actually lower blood cholesterol.

Choosing Heart-Healthy Foods

Foods are categorized here by how heavily they're packed with calories—how calorie dense they are compared with other foods—high, medium or low. The upper half of this chart shows common foods in the typical American diet, all coded to indicate those that are especially high in saturated fat: **SF**; cholesterol: **C**; salt: **SA**; and sugar: **SU**. The lower half shows more healthful alternatives.

Usual Food Pattern for United States

High Calorie Density	Medium Calorie Density	Low Calorie Density
Commercial baked goods: **SF; C; SA; SU**	Buttermilk: **SF; C; SA**	Bouillon: **SA**
Bacon: **SF; C; SA**	Egg yolk: **SF; C**	Canned vegetable juice: **SA**
Frankfurter: **SF; C; SA**	Whole milk: **SF; C**	Consommé: **SA**
Ham, sausage: **SF; C; SA**	Granola with added salt and sugar: **SA; SU**	Melba toast: **SA**
Luncheon meat: **SF; C; SA**	Shellfish: **C**	Most canned vegetables: **SA**
Most regular cheeses: **SF; C; SA**	Dehydrated potatoes: **SA**	Pickles: **SA**
Ice cream: **SF; C; SU**	Most canned soups: **SA**	Salted popcorn: **SA**
Organ meat: **SF; C**	Most canned tuna: **SA**	Sauerkraut: **SA**
Red meat: **SF; C**	Saltines: **SA**	
Potato chips: **SA**	Turkey franks: **SA**	
Salted nuts: **SA**	Most soft drinks: **SU**	
Palm oil, coconut oil: **SF**		
Candy: **SU**		
Fruit in heavy syrup: **SU**		

Healthier Food Pattern

High Calorie Density	Medium Calorie Density	Low Calorie Density
Avocado	Brown rice	Artichokes
No-salt peanut butter	Corn	Beets
Sesame butter	Egg whites	Broccoli
Soft margarine	Fresh or dried fruit	Brussels sprouts
Sunflower seeds	Fresh fish	Cabbage
Unsalted nuts	Fruit juice with pulp	Carrots
Vegetable oils, except palm and coconut	Granola without salt or sugar	Cauliflower
	Legumes (beans, lentils, peas)	Celery
	Lightly milled or whole-grain breads	Chard
	Low-fat cottage cheese	Cucumbers
	Nonfat milk	Fresh vegetable juice
	Pasta	Green beans
	Potatoes	Lettuce
	Shredded wheat	Mushrooms
	Sweet potatoes	Spinach
	Turkey	Squash
		Tomatoes

SOURCE: Adapted from *The American Way of Life Need Not Be Hazardous to Your Health* by John W. Farquhar (New York: W. W. Norton & Co., 1979).

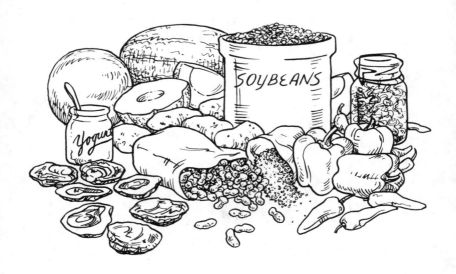

The Three-Phase Program for a Healthier Heart

Taken together, all of these heart-saving dietary factors constitute the best "anti-heart-attack" diet science can devise. Unfortunately, such a diet goes against the grain of the average American way of eating. So the question is, can you really change the entrenched eating habits of a lifetime?

Judging from research at Stanford and elsewhere, the answer has to be yes. But you can't—and shouldn't—do it overnight. Overnight dietary changes are likely to be temporary. Gradual changes are apt to stick with you.

That is the reason we are offering a three-phase program for slow but steady progress toward heart-healthy eating. Each phase can last as long as a year, depending on how easy you find each one, and can drastically lower your risk of heart disease.

You can see for yourself what the phased changes can do to your coronary risk by periodically retaking the risk test on pages 70 to 73.

Following are the recommended eating patterns for each phase. But before you embark on Phase I, consider:

- In this program you neither have to give up all your favorite foods nor abruptly cut anything from your diet. You will, however, explore and enjoy new flavors.
- You increase your chances of success if you concentrate on one or two dietary problems at a time. You could, for example, work on lowering your intake of fat, cholesterol and sugar for the first two or three months, then integrate efforts to cut back on salt over the next two months—all the while slowly boosting your intake of low-calorie, high-fiber carbohydrates.
- If you're the only one in your family trying out new eating patterns, you'll probably revert to your old ways in no time. Modifying dietary habits should be a family affair—and it easily can be when the changes happen slowly and comfortably.

Phase I. This is your first controlled step away from the average American diet—an easy transition in which you keep most of your old food habits but substitute for foods highest in salt, sugar, saturated fat and cholesterol. (The table on pages 64 and 65 will help you identify the culprit foods.) In this stage you can reduce your fat intake from the United States average of 40 percent of total calories to 30 percent and set a goal of losing perhaps one-third of any excess weight. Don't go on to Phase II until you're comfortable with all of the following changes:

1. Reduce by one-half the number of weekly servings of whole milk, ice cream, cheese (except low-fat varieties) and fatty meats (beef, lamb, bacon, spareribs, sausage and luncheon meats). In their place, substitute fish, poultry and complex carbohydrate foods.
2. Switch from ice cream to ice milk, from whole to nonfat milk and from regular to nonfat yogurt.
3. Trim the fat off meat and broil or roast the meat instead of frying it.
4. Rarely, if ever, eat organ meats like liver, sweetbreads and brains.
5. Switch from butter or hard margarine to soft tub margarine and use unhydrogenated vegetable oil instead of lard or shortening.

6. Cut back on egg yolks to no more than four a week, but use egg whites liberally.
7. Switch from peanut butter made with hydrogenated fat to peanut butter without hydrogenated fat.
8. Cut back on fast foods, processed or convenience foods and commercial baked goods.
9. Cut your consumption of sugar-sweetened soft drinks in half. (Limit yourself to two or three a week. The average is five 12-ounce servings per week.) Slowly wean yourself off sugar in your coffee or tea. Switch from fruit canned in heavy syrup to fruit canned in light syrup, and for one-third of your desserts substitute fruit for pastry, cake, pie and other sweets.
10. Drastically reduce your intake of high-salt foods such as bacon, ham, sausage, frankfurters, luncheon meats, sauerkraut, salted nuts, pickles and salted snack foods. Gradually eliminate the use of salt at the table and cut the use of salt in cooking by two-thirds. Use salt substitutes to help you make the transition, and experiment with spices, herbs, lemon, wine and vinegar.
11. Increase your intake of whole fruits and vegetables and lightly milled or whole grains (for example, whole wheat bread, cracked wheat, rolled oats, bulgur, brown rice and rye).

Phase II.   At least 16 national and international advisory bodies (including the American Heart Association and the U.S. Senate Select Committee on Nutrition and Human Needs) have recommended dietary changes that approximate those in Phase II. This stage will allow you to further reduce your intake of dietary "artery blockers," to rein in your fat intake to about 25 percent of total calories and to reduce your risk-quiz score to one point for each of the food-related risks (weight, blood pressure and cholesterol). It's a time for culinary experiments in heart-healthy ethnic cuisine—Middle Eastern, Mediterranean, Mexican, Indian—and in meatless (or almost meatless) meals.

1. Reduce overall servings of red meat, egg yolks, ice cream, cheese (except low-fat varieties) and whole milk to eight per week. Restrict even further your intake of processed and convenience foods high in saturated fats.
2. Limit sugar-sweetened soft drinks to rare occasions, use

water-packed canned fruit instead of fruit in light syrup and substitute fruit for two-thirds of all your desserts.

3. Eliminate almost all salt when cooking vegetables and substitute other seasonings—but not high-sodium flavorings like celery salt, onion salt, steak sauce and soy sauce. Use the no-salt-added versions of peanut butter, ketchup, canned vegetables, canned tuna fish and other store-bought foods.

4. Increase your intake of whole grain breads, high-fiber cereals and whole fruits and vegetables to at least five servings of such foods per day. Make sure that at least half the fruit juices you drink contain pulp.

Phase III.   Some of you may want to stay in Phase II indefinitely, and that's fine. It's a safe haven for the heart. But you can reduce your risk even more by venturing into Phase III, an optimal eating plan not only for deterring heart disease but also for greatly decreasing your chances of getting hemorrhoids, type II diabetes, (that is, the more prevalent, non-insulin-dependent diabetes that tends to develop later in life), diseases associated with obesity, dental problems and cancer of the colon, rectum and breast. This stage allows you to drop your fat intake to 20 percent of calories (about half the American average), raise your intake of complex carbohydrates to 55 percent of calories and reduce your risk-quiz score on food-related risks to rock bottom— a healthy zero.

1. Reduce the overall number of servings of red meat, egg yolks, ice cream, cheese (except for low-fat types) and whole milk to five a week. Watch for hidden sources of saturated fat in restaurant fare and convenience foods.

2. Make fruit and nuts your main source of desserts. For breakfast, lunch and snacks, experiment with combinations of fresh fruit, nuts and whole grain cereals. Ban table sugar and use small amounts of honey instead.

3. Use almost no salt in all cooking and keep looking for ways to avoid excess salt in store-bought foods.

4. Each day, eat at least seven servings of fruit, vegetables, whole grain cereals (like brown rice, whole wheat and bulgur) and legumes of all kinds. Discover the multitude of existing tasty recipes using these foods.

Weighing Less, Living Longer

A lot of people think that the biggest problem with overweight is that it makes you look and feel bad. But these are small worries next to its true supreme drawback: It can kill you. Carrying around excess flab can overwork your heart, raise your blood pressure and cholesterol and increase your chances of getting diabetes, which is a coronary risk factor in itself.

Assess Your Risk of Heart Attack and Stroke

Your diet, of course, is one of the major factors determining your health and your risk of having heart trouble. Getting enough exercise, not smoking cigarettes and reducing stress also help lower the risk. In 60 seconds you can have a rough estimate of your chances of developing serious heart problems, simply by taking the risk quiz on pages 72 and 73. It lists the six primary risk factors of heart disease, each with a possible score of 0 to 4. Go through each risk factor and circle the score that applies to you, then add up all the numbers for a total score. The lower your total score, the lower your estimated risk. Maximum total score is 24 points; the American average is an unhealthy 14. Here's what your total score means:

21 to 24 points—Your probability of having a premature heart attack or stroke is about four or five times the U.S. average. Action is urgent. Try to drop four points within a month and three more within six months.

17 to 20 points—Your chance of having a heart attack or stroke is about twice the U.S. average. Take action now. Try to drop four points within six months.

13 to 16 points—This is close to the U.S. average, a risky place to be. With careful planning you can shave five or six points off your total score within a year.

About 80 to 90 percent of adult Americans are above their ideal weight, which means that in the United States, flab is typical—but it certainly isn't normal. On the average, for example, American men are 20 to 30 pounds heavier than men of the same age and height in many other countries. Americans typically—but abnormally—gain weight after age 20. In nations without Western styles of eating and sedentary living, adults generally *lose* pounds as they age due to normal loss of muscle mass in the aging process.

(continued on page 74)

9 to 12 points—The likelihood of your having a heart attack or stroke is about half the U.S. average. Most people with a total score between 13 and 20 can easily reach this rating in a year, and you can cut four to six points off this rating in the same amount of time.

5 to 8 points—Your probability of heart attack or stroke is about a quarter of the U.S. average. A lot of people can achieve this goal in one or two years.

0 to 4 points—Your chances of heart attack or stroke are very low, about one-tenth of the U.S. average for the 35-to-65 age-group. This level, which can take three to four years for the average person to reach, requires plenty of effort and lots of family support.

Note: If you're a woman, your ideal weight equals (your height in inches times 3.5) minus 108. If you're a man, your ideal weight equals (your height in inches times 4) minus 128. (This formula works best for people with average builds. People with small or large frames may need to refer to standard weight charts.) If all your exercise is competitive, add one point to your total risk score. If your intake of fiber is high (if you eat almost no sugar but lots of fruits, vegetables and whole grains), subtract one point.

If you're a woman taking estrogen or birth control pills, add one point if your total risk score is 12 or below, two points if your total risk score is 13 or above.

Risk Factor	Increasing Risk				
Smoking Cigarettes Score	None 0	Up to 9/day 1	10 to 24/day 2	25 to 34/day 3	35 or more/day 4
Body Weight Score	Ideal weight 0	Up to 9 lb. excess 1	10 to 19 lb. excess 2	20 to 29 lb. excess 3	30 or more lb. excess 4
Salt Intake	⅓ avg. No added salt, no convenience foods	⅓ avg. No use of salt at table, little use of high-salt foods	U.S. avg. Salt in cooking, some salt at table	Above avg. Frequent salt at table	Far above avg. Frequent use of salty foods
Or if known, **Blood Pressure Upper Reading** Score	Less than 110 0	110-129 1	130-139 2	140-149 3	150 or over 4
Saturated Fat and Cholesterol Intake	⅓ avg. Almost total vegetarian; rare egg yolk, butterfat and lean meat	⅓ avg. 2 meatless days/wk., no whole milk products, lean meat only	½ avg. Meat (mostly lean), eggs, cheese 12 times/wk.; nonfat milk only	U.S. avg. Meat, cheese, eggs, whole milk 24 times/wk.	Above avg. Meat, cheese, eggs, whole milk over 24 times/wk.
Or if known, **Blood Cholesterol Level** Score	Less than 150 0	150-169 1	170-199 2	200-219 3	220 or over 4

Exercise	Vigorous exercise 4 or more times/wk., 20 min. each or Brisk walking 5 times/wk., 45 min. each	Vigorous exercise 3 times/wk., 20 min. each or Brisk walking 3 times/wk., 30 min. each	Vigorous exercise 1 or 2 times/wk., 20 min. each or Brisk walking 2 times/wk., 30 min. each	U.S. avg. Occasional exercise or Normal walking 2½ to 4½ miles daily	Below avg. Rare exercise or Normal walking less than 2½ miles daily
Score	0	1	2	3	4
Stress	Rarely tense or anxious or Yoga, meditation, or equivalent 20 min. 2 times/day	Calmer than avg., feel tense about 3 times/wk.	U.S. avg. Feel tense or anxious 2 or 3 times/day, frequent anger or hurried feelings	Tense, usually rushed, occasional tranquilizer	Extremely tense, take tranquilizers 5 or more times/wk.
Score	0	1	2	3	4

SOURCE: Adapted from *The American Way of Life Need Not Be Hazardous to Your Health* by John W. Farquhar (New York: W. W. Norton & Co., 1979).

But it's not as though Americans haven't been trying to fight fat. The popular cycle of gaining, losing and regaining weight—the rhythm method of girth control—is an American institution. It's fueled by generations of fad diets and quick fixes and has left behind a lot of frustrated, cynical dieters.

"Fad diets usually lead to weight loss that's rapidly regained," says C. Barr Taylor, M.D., a psychiatrist who conducts weight-control studies at Stanford. "This does more harm than good. Often after going off one of these diets, the weight piles on faster than before. And some diets are so extreme that they skimp on nutrition to get rid of extra pounds."

The trouble with weight-loss diets, fad or not, is that they're just diets, just eating patterns—they don't change underlying behavior that leads to weight gain, and they don't have the important element of exercise. Permanent weight loss almost always means slowly, and thus painlessly, altering some lifestyle habits as you fine-tune your menus. And it means exercising to accelerate the loss of fat, to avoid the loss of muscle tissue that dieting by itself causes, to firm up your body as you drop weight, to speed up your metabolism so you can burn more calories even when you're at rest and—believe it or not—to allow you to eat more and still lose weight.

So Stanford researchers suggest an approach that covers all the bases—diet, behavior and exercise—and is as individual as you are. Based on their research and experience helping people lose unwanted pounds, we recommend the following:

Set reasonable goals.   Ultimately, you want to get back to your ideal weight, but simply reducing enough to ease into a safer risk category would be an accomplishment. Whatever your target weight is, give yourself plenty of time to get there. Losing just ten pounds a year can be a big accomplishment. The rule of thumb: Don't try to drop more than one or two pounds a week.

Eat three meals a day (including breakfast).   In those meals include more foods low in fat and sugar but high in complex carbohydrates, fiber, vitamins and minerals. In other words, embark on an eating plan like Phase I, easing toward Phases II and III. If you prefer to keep better track of calories, use the table on pages 64 and 65. It tells you which foods are packed with calories (HCD, or high calorie density, foods) and which aren't. The table is a reasonable substitute for more cumbersome calorie-counting charts and can help you systematically cut down on a lot of fattening foods. For example, if you know the number of HCD foods you eat each day (the American average is 15), you can plan gradual cutbacks from week to week.

Exercise regularly.   If you don't exercise, your body is more likely to adjust to any cutback in calorie intake and hold onto its pockets of fat. Slowly work into regular aerobic workouts and increase your level of daily activity—take stairs instead of elevators, walk or bicycle to work, park at the far end of the parking lot, do some gardening, walk to lunch or try your own method of burning calories.

Don't rely on will power.   Build commitment. Make a two-week contract with yourself to cut down on certain fattening foods, or work out so many times a week, or whatever. Fulfill that contract and draw up another, then another. Ask a friend or spouse to help you monitor your progress and give moral support. If you do better in groups, join a health club, gym or weight-loss organization.

Alter the behaviors that increase your chances of failure.   Eat slowly, savoring completely, putting your fork down between mouthfuls and spending 20 to 25 minutes on each meal; eat only in the kitchen or dining room and only because it's time to eat, not because you're bored or stressed or habit-prone; plan to eat two low-calorie snacks daily, one at midmorning and the other at midafternoon, concentrating only on the food for ten minutes; at mealtime, put food out of sight after first helpings; if you ban a food from your diet, keep it out of the house; avoid rigid, perfectionistic thinking that leads to disappointment ("I'll never eat another cookie as long as I live."); don't be too hard on yourself for occasionally deviating from your program ("I have no will power, so I might as well stop trying.").

Reward yourself for reaching goals.   Buy yourself a present, do something you love to do (no gorging on high-calorie foods!), tell yourself you're terrific.

Foods to Help Lower Your Blood Pressure for Life

You begin your day with a juicy half-moon of cantaloupe, a glass of freshly squeezed orange juice and a bowl of bran cereal with half a cup of skim milk.

Lunch is broiled mackerel, parsley potatoes and a side salad of watercress, carrot medallions and almonds, tossed with your own dressing made of fresh garlic in corn oil and apple cider vinegar.

In midafternoon, you calm your rumbling stomach with a cup of low-fat yogurt into which you've sliced half a banana.

For dinner, you whip up a luscious casserole of brown rice, onions, broccoli, cashews and melted part-skim mozzarella, lightly spiced with garlic.

If you have high blood pressure, theoretically you've just done everything right. Your one day's menu contains every nutrient known to *lower* blood pressure. Today, medical research has uncovered a way to fight hypertension that's more positive than just avoiding salt and saturated fat. There are actually foods you can eat more of that help you win this often-deadly numbers game.

And if you didn't know already, high blood pressure can be deadly. According to Michael Rees, M.D., author of *The Complete Family Guide to Living with High Blood Pressure,* hypertension is a major cause of diseases of the heart, brain, kidneys and eyes. In fact, hypertension is the single most important cause of strokes and is the cause of an estimated one-third of all heart disease. Some 60 million Americans have blood pressure that is too high, blood pressure that just might respond to some dietary fine-tuning. They might want to start with this menu.

Potassium-Rich Foods Offer Protection

Cantaloupe, winter squash, potatoes, broccoli, orange juice, some fresh fruits and milk contain hefty amounts of potassium. And the fact is, how much potassium you have in your diet may be just as important as how little sodium you eat. Studies of vegetarians, who tend to have lower blood pressure than meat eaters, found that their sodium intake was no different from that of hypertensives, but their potassium intake was significantly higher.

A group of scientists in Israel looked at the eating habits of 98 vegetarians whose average age was 60 and compared them with a similar group of meat eaters. What they found was a very low prevalence of hypertension—only 2 percent—among the vegetarians, although they lived in an adult population where the expected prevalence was 20 to 25 percent. The vegetarians ate as much salt as their neighbors and had the same genetic predisposition to developing hypertension. But they didn't. The researchers concluded that it was their potassium-rich diet of vegetables, fruits and nuts that kept them from developing hypertension.

Just how does potassium protect the body from hypertension, even when sodium intake isn't restricted? No one really knows, although there are a number of theories. For one, potassium is an effective diuretic—and has been used as one for nearly four centuries. But in addition to helping the body rid itself of water, potassium also helps slough off sodium, an effect called natriuresis. Potassium also appears to act on several important physiological systems that regulate blood pressure and control the workings of the vascular system.

In both animal and human studies, potassium seems to have little effect on people whose blood pressure is normal. But it can produce a significant drop in both systolic (representing blood pressure during heart muscle contractions) and diastolic (representing blood pressure during the relaxation phase of a heartbeat) pressures of hypertensives.

And there may be one group of people for whom potassium is literally a shield against the ravages of excess sodium. According to George R. Meneely, M.D., emeritus professor of medicine at Louisiana State University School of Medicine, there may be "a substantial fraction of the population worldwide, including primitive societies, who develop elevation of the blood pressure if they eat more than four grams of sodium as sodium chloride [normal table salt] a day.

"There is extensive animal evidence," says Dr. Meneely, "that the hypertensogenic [hypertension-causing] effect of excess sodium is counteracted by extra dietary potassium. There is pretty good literature on its effect in humans, too."

For anyone who wants to increase his or her dietary potassium, here's a cooking tip from a group of Swedish scientists: To avoid potassium loss in cooking, steam rather than boil vegetables. When doctors at a Swedish hospital tested the two cooking methods with potatoes, a rich source of potassium, they discovered that boiled potatoes lost 10 to 50 percent of their potassium, while steamed potatoes lost only 3 to 6 percent. They had similar results with carrots, beans and peas.

A Calcium Bounty in Your Refrigerator

Dairy products, leafy green vegetables like kale and watercress, and nuts contain calcium. And if you've been scrupulous about cutting sodium out of your diet, you may be cutting out calcium, too. There's a convincing amount of evidence from all corners of the world indicating that calcium can lower your blood pressure. Unfortunately, the best sources of calcium—dairy products—also have a fair amount of sodium. A two-ounce serving of Swiss cheese contains 544 milligrams of calcium (the Recommended Dietary Allowance is 800 milligrams), but there's a hefty 148 milligrams of sodium in there, too. But the evidence is too overwhelming in favor of calcium as an antidote to hypertension for anyone to give up milk and cheese entirely.

Consider, for example, a study of 82 percent of the adult residents of Rancho Bernardo, an upper middle-class community in Southern California. What separated the male hypertensives from the people with normal blood pressure, according to researchers at the University of California at San Diego, was milk. Milk consumption was lower in borderline, untreated and treated hypertensives.

In an even larger study, involving 20,749 people across the country, calcium was the only one of 17 nutrients evaluated that differed in the hypertensives. Those people with high blood pressure consumed 18 percent less calcium.

That figure alarms researcher David McCarron, M.D., of the division of nephrology and hypertension at the Oregon Health Sciences University in Portland. He conducted that particular study—and several others linking calcium and blood pressure—and he's convinced that a good hypertensive diet has to contain dairy products, even though they contain sodium and cholesterol.

"If you have to, switch to low-sodium or low-cholesterol cheeses, which are an excellent source of calcium and low in saturated fatty acids," he says. "If you don't have a cholesterol problem and you're near your ideal body weight, you don't necessarily have to worry about the cholesterol."

As for sodium, Dr. McCarron's work indicates that calcium may actually negate the harmful effects of salt on the system. An increased calcium load tends to facilitate the body's excretion of sodium, he notes.

Calcium works on blood pressure in another way—by relaxing the blood vessels. "You'll rarely hear a doctor say that, because the most doctors are ever taught in medical school is that calcium makes blood vessels contract," he says. "When blood vessels contract, blood pressure goes up. But calcium actually regulates contraction *and* relaxation of the blood vessels."

But one of the most interesting things to come out of Dr. McCarron's research is not how calcium works alone to lower blood pressure but how it works with potassium, sodium and magnesium to regulate pressure. "It's the proportions of these minerals in the body that seem to be the most important thing," says Dr. McCarron. "The possibility exists that the more you want to eat of one, the more you'd better eat of the others. We, of course, consider calcium the most important. But if you're not taking in enough sodium, potassium and magnesium, the probability is that you're not getting enough calcium either."

And, not coincidentally, the foods that are abundant in one tend to be abundant in the others.

Magnesium As a Partner in Health

Nuts, brown rice, molasses, milk, wheat germ, bananas, potatoes and soy products provide magnesium. Inadequate dietary magnesium has been shown to increase blood pressure in both animals and humans. Though the exact mechanism isn't known, there is some indication that magnesium exerts its pressure-lowering effect by regulating the entry and exit of calcium in the smooth muscle cells of the vascular system. Together, the two minerals produce the regular contraction and relaxation of blood vessels.

In a test involving untreated, newly diagnosed hypertensives, Dr. McCarron found that they consumed less calcium and magnesium than members of a similar group whose blood pressure was normal. Sodium intake didn't seem to matter.

"The interaction of magnesium and calcium gives the calcium the ability to get where it has to in a cell," says Dr. McCarron. "Magnesium facilitates calcium getting to the right place where it can have this relaxing effect."

Some Fats Are Good for Your Blood Pressure

In a pilot study of healthy people in Italy, Finland and the United States, researchers discovered that the level of dietary linoleic acid—polyunsaturated fats derived from plant foods—was associated with incidence of high blood pressure. There were more hypertensives among the Finnish population than among the Italians and Americans. The Finns consumed more saturated and less polyunsaturated fats than the others.

When a group of Finns aged 40 to 50 were placed on a low-fat diet high in polyunsaturated fats and low in saturated fats, even when salt consumption wasn't reduced, blood pressure dropped significantly. When they returned to their old eating habits, their old blood pressure returned, too.

What's the magic? James M. Iacono, Ph.D., and other researchers at the U.S. Department of Agriculture Western Human Nutrition Research Center in San Francisco have one theory. They believe poly-unsaturated fats lower blood pressure because, when they're metabolized by the body, they yield a substance that is essential for making prostaglandins. These are fatty acids that seem to control pressure by aiding in the sloughing off of water and salt from the kidneys.

The Role of Fish

As discussed in chapter 2, mackerel and other marine fish are high in eicosapentanoic acid, one of the omega-3 fatty acids. Tests in Germany involving 15 volunteers on a mackerel diet provided some heartening results. After only two weeks, serum triglycerides and total cholesterol dropped significantly, mirrored by "markedly lower" systolic and diastolic blood pressures.

The Germans didn't simply pull mackerel out of their hats. They were attempting to approximate the diet of Greenland Eskimos and Japanese fishermen, who enjoy a very low incidence of cardiovascular disease. They key appears to be the omega-3 fatty acids found in many fish.

Another study tested the effects of cod-liver oil, which also contains omega-3 fatty acids, on the Western diet. A group of volunteers added three tablespoons of cod-liver oil a day to their normal diet and wound up with lower blood pressure.

The Move to Include More Fiber

Bran, fresh fruits and vegetables, beans and whole grain breads supply fiber. There are some early indications from recent tests that plant fiber can significantly lower blood pressure, though precisely why is still a mystery.

Researcher James W. Anderson, M.D., of the Veterans Administration Medical Center in Lexington, Kentucky, placed 12 diabetic men on a 14-day diet containing more than three times the dietary fiber (and fat) of a control group's diet. Average blood pressure dropped 10 percent. In patients whose blood pressure had been normal, systolic pressure was 8 percent lower, and the diastolic figure dropped 10 percent.

The news was even better for the men who had high blood pressure to begin with. Their systolic pressure dropped by 11 percent, and diastolic pressure was 10 percent lower.

Dr. Anderson was pleased with his results, but he's not sure why he got them.

"My strongest hunch is that it's related to certain changes in insulin. The patients' insulin needs were low on the high-fiber diet. There's a lot of evidence that insulin contributes to high blood pressure. It's basically a salt-retentive hormone. We also reported a small increase in sodium loss in feces. I didn't think at the time it was meaningful, but thinking about it later, having two different mechanisms working together like that—the insulin and the sodium excretion— you can get a synergistic effect."

What makes the results even more significant is that salt use was not restricted during the diet. "In fact," says Dr. Anderson, "there was a 50 percent increase in sodium intake. But potassium also went up, so the sodium/potassium ratio stayed the same."

What's on Your Breath
Needn't Worry Your Heart

The old wives were right. Their tale of onions lowering blood pressure was on target—they do. What the old wives didn't know was why. According to Moses Attrep, Jr., Ph.D., a chemist at East Texas State University, it may be due to a hormonelike substance he isolated in yellow onions called prostaglandin A_1, which also occurs in the human kidney. When injected into humans and animals, prostaglandin A_1 lowers blood pressure, at least for brief periods.

The old wives were right about garlic, too. The Japanese and Chinese have used garlic to lower blood pressure for centuries. Its effect is possibly similar to that of onions, since it might also contain prostaglandins. Dr. Attrep is working on an answer to the garlic riddle, too.

The Cancer-Prevention Diet

Many of us have lived with a feeling of helplessness about cancer for so long that it's hard to change our thinking. But a massive body of research now refutes the long-held belief that we are at the mercy of cancer; it shows instead that we can prevent it.

How much of an impact could we have if we all practiced prevention?

"If it were possible that we could carry it out ideally, as much as 80 to 85 percent of all cancers today might not occur," says Charles A. LeMaistre, M.D., president of the American Cancer Society. "For too long we have regarded curing cancer as the dominant factor in its relationship with man. Now preventing this disease is becoming more and more realistic."

By avoiding the things known to cause cancer and incorporating into our lives factors that protect against it, we can reduce our risk of developing the disease.

"In some areas, the information is now so complete that it's unequivocal, such as the causal role of smoking in the development of cancer," says Dr. LeMaistre, who is also president of the University of

Texas's M. D. Anderson Hospital and Tumor Institute in Houston. "In other areas, such as diet and nutrition, information is not yet complete, but it is sufficient to take action."

Eight Ways to Protect Yourself

The following steps summarize what we can do, and they are recommended by the American Cancer Society. They will also contribute to a healthier life in general.

1. Eat more high-fiber foods.   These include whole grains, fruits and vegetables. There is a lot of evidence that colon cancer is less common in populations whose diet is high in fiber. In a study comparing Finnish and Danish people, for example, colon cancer was much lower among the Finns. The diets of the two groups are similar, except that the Finns eat large amounts of high-fiber, whole grain rye bread, while the Danes have a low-fiber diet.

Fiber may work by hastening the travel time of fecal matter through the bowel, so that carcinogens (cancer-causing substances) are whisked away before they can do their damage. Another theory is that by increasing the bulk of the stool, fiber dilutes the concentration of carcinogens.

2. Eat more foods rich in vitamin A.   Spinach, carrots, sweet potatoes and apricots are good examples. They may help protect you against cancers of the lung, esophagus and larynx. In a major study, Norwegian men whose intake of vitamin A was above average had less than half the rate of lung cancer of men whose intake of the vitamin was below average.

Right now it's unclear whether the effects are due to vitamin A itself or a precursor of vitamin A called beta-carotene, a pigment found in plants. The emphasis now is on the naturally occurring pigment, because the precursors of vitamin A are the most probable agents that have this effect.

Beta-carotene is found in dark green and deep yellow vegetables and in deep yellow fruits.

3. Get plenty of vitamin C.   Studies indicate that people whose diets are rich in vitamin C are less likely to get cancer, particularly cancer of the stomach and esophagus.

We know that vitamin C can inhibit the formation of nitrosamines, cancer-causing chemicals, in the stomach. That may be how it protects against cancer.

Fruits and vegetables, particularly oranges, grapefruit, green peppers, broccoli, tomatoes and potatoes, are good sources of the vitamin.

4. Eat more cabbage-family vegetables. Broccoli, brussels sprouts, cabbage, cauliflower, kale and kohlrabi are close relatives. Studies in large groups of people have suggested that consuming these vegetables, also called cruciferous vegetables, may reduce the risk of cancer, particularly cancer of the gastrointestinal and respiratory tracts. And tests in laboratory animals reveal that cruciferous vegetables may be highly effective in preventing chemically induced cancer.

What is it about these foods that is protective? "We have to look upon these vegetables as a source of vitamins A and C and fiber, but there are other possibilities under investigation," Dr. LeMaistre notes.

5. Trim fat from your diet. Laboratory studies and studies in humans point out that excessive fat intake increases the chance of developing cancers of the breast, colon and prostate. And it's not just one kind of fat that's a problem—both saturated and unsaturated fats, whether of plant or animal origin, have been found to enhance cancer growth when eaten in excess.

The National Academy of Sciences recommends that we decrease the amount of fat in our diet to 30 percent of the total calories we eat (Americans currently consume about 40 percent of total calories as fat).

You can cut your fat intake by using less fats and oils in cooking and by switching to lean meat and fish and low-fat dairy products.

6. Control your weight. "The long-standing and repeated observation that obesity is correlated with cancer is sufficiently substantiated to take action," says Dr. LeMaistre. In one massive study conducted by the American Cancer Society over 12 years, researchers found an increased incidence of cancers of the uterus, gallbladder, breast, colon, kidney and stomach in obese people. In that study, women and men who were 40 percent or more overweight had a 55 and 33 percent greater risk of cancer, respectively, than people of normal weight.

Regular exercise and lower calorie intake can help you avoid gaining weight. It's advisable to check with your doctor before embarking on a special diet or strenuous exercise routine, though.

7. Avoid salt-cured, smoked and nitrite-cured foods.
These include ham, bacon, hot dogs and salt-cured or smoked fish. Cancers of the esophagus and stomach are common in countries where large quantities of these foods are eaten.

Smoked foods absorb some of the tars from the smoke they're cured with. The tars contain cancer-causing chemicals similar to those in tobacco smoke. There is also good evidence that nitrate and nitrite can enhance the formation of nitrosamines in our food and in our digestive tract.

8. Go easy on alcohol.
Heavy drinkers, especially those who also smoke, are at very high risk for cancers of the mouth and throat. Your risk of liver cancer also increases if you drink a lot.

In addition to eating a healthier diet, the following steps will further decrease your risk of getting cancer: Don't smoke cigarettes, shield yourself from the sun and avoid excessive x-rays, estrogen and exposure at work to harmful chemicals and fibers such as asbestos. Also, early detection methods such as sigmoidoscopy, Pap tests and breast exams can catch any cancer that does sneak up when there's still a very good chance of curing it.

Putting It All Together

Experts agree that it's your total diet that keeps you on target healthwise. This handy chart sums up which foods spell good health when eaten frequently and which foods should be eaten only occasionally or seldom. We hope you'll find this at-a-glance nutrition guide useful when grocery shopping for your family.

The Good-Health Diet Plan

Eat Frequently	Eat Occasionally	Eat Seldom
Dairy foods	**Dairy foods**	**Dairy foods**
Low-fat yogurt (plain)	Swiss cheese	Ice cream
Skim milk	Mozzarella (part skim)	Sherbet
	Gruyere cheese	
	Gouda cheese	
	American cheese	

(continued)

The Good-Health Diet Plan—*Continued*

Eat Frequently	Eat Occasionally	Eat Seldom
Meat, fish, poultry, eggs	**Meat, fish, poultry, eggs**	**Meat, fish, poultry, eggs**
Swordfish*	Chicken (with skin)	Sturgeon (smoked)
Salmon*	Turkey (with skin)	Anchovies
Trout*	Round steak	Fish sticks
Halibut*	Chuck roast	Duck
Shrimp*	Porterhouse steak	Poultry (fried)
Chicken (skinned)	Flank steak	Liver
Turkey (skinned)	Lean ground beef	Sirloin steak
	Leg of lamb	Club steak
Vegetables	Rump roast (choice)	Lamb ribs
	Veat cutlet	Bologna
Red peppers	Veal loin	Salami
Kale and spinach	Ham	Bacon
Broccoli	Pork chops	Hash
Acorn squash	Pork roast	Sausage
Lima beans		Eggs (fried)
Carrots	**Grains, cereals**	Fish (fried)
Brussels sprouts		
Navy beans	Crackers	**Vegetables**
Cauliflower	Pretzels	
Garlic		Vegetables in cream
	Nuts, seeds	sauce
Fruits		Fried vegetables
	Sunflower seeds	
Apricots (dried)	Almonds	**Fruits**
Blackberries	Pumpkin seeds	
Raspberries	Sesame seeds	Fruit packed in heavy
Strawberries	Peanuts (raw or roasted)	syrup
Cantaloupes	Cashews	Fruit drinks
Bananas	Peanut butter	Fruit leather
Grains, cereals		**Grains, cereals**
Bran		Cookies
Amaranth		
Millet		

SOURCE: Prepared in cooperation with Annette B. Natow, Ph.D., R.D., and Jo-Ann Heslin, M.A., R.D.

*Broiled, poached, steamed or baked.